SUPER *foods*
FOR CHILDREN

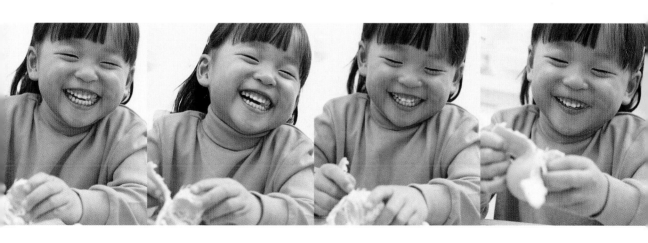

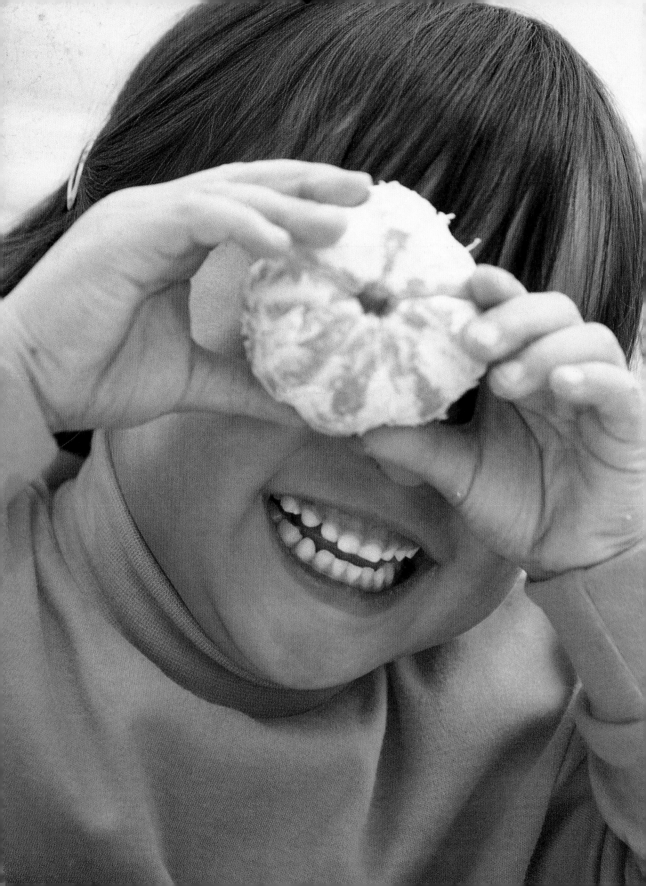

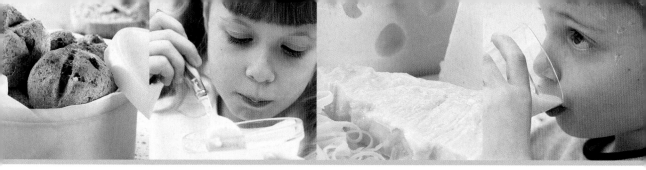

SUPER *foods*
FOR CHILDREN

michael van straten
& barbara griggs

US medical editor: Thomas G. Sherman, PhD

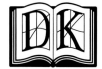

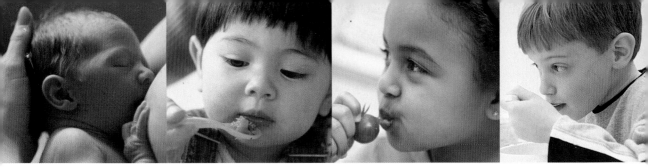

contents

nutrition without numbers   6

Nailing the facts behind food labels and manufacturers' slogans: how to choose foods that look good, taste good, and greatly benefit children – and how to avoid foods that don't.

nutrition on a plate   10

The basics of nutrition explained, with a guide to those foods that contain valuable amounts of the essential nutrients.

carbohydrates 12 ★ protein 15 ★ fats 16 ★ minerals 18 ★ vitamins & antioxidants 20 ★ organic foods 22

superfoods   24

Over 130 top foods and groups of foods that form the building blocks of healthy eating for children, with a hard look at foods to avoid.

super vegetables 26 ★ super salads 31 ★ super fruits 34 ★ super legumes 42 ★ super nuts & seeds 44 ★ super grains 47 ★ super meat 52 ★ super poultry 54 ★ super fish 56 ★ super dairy foods 58 ★ super fats 62 ★ herbs & spices 64 ★ the danger foods 66

meals for every age group   70

An explanation of the nutritional needs at each stage of childhood, with profiles of superfoods and danger foods, and weekly menu plans based on the book's recipes.

enjoying good food 72 ★ healthy babies from day one 74 ★ breast-feeding & baby meals 78 ★ hungry toddlers 84 ★ pre-school years 88 ★ off to school 92 ★ the years of growth 96 ★ turbulent teens 100 ★ vegetarian children 104

family kitchen   108

Constructive tips on how parents and children can make the best use of the family kitchen and on safe hygiene and food preparation.

what you need 110 ★ hygiene in the kitchen 114

superfood recipes   116

Over 160 recipes, using the superfoods, for appetizing dishes. Includes ideas for instant snacks and what to have in the refrigerator.

about the recipes 118 ★ big breakfasts 120 ★ super soups 128 ★ tasty lunches 136 ★ snacks & light meals 150 ★ satisfying suppers 164 ★ desserts 186 ★ delicious drinks 192 ★ instant good food 196

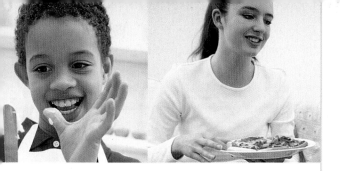

LONDON, NEW YORK, SYDNEY, DELHI, PARIS,
MUNICH and JOHANNESBURG

*This book is dedicated
to the memory of
Jason and Ninka*

Senior Managing Art Editor Lynne Brown
Project Editor Janice Anderson
Art Editor Glenda Fisher
Designer Bernhard Koppmeyer
Food Photography Simon Smith, Trish Gant
Model Photography Vanessa Davies
DTP Designer Karen Constanti
Production Controller Melissa Allsopp
US Editor Barbara Minton
US DTP Tracy McCord
US Medical Editor Thomas G. Sherman, PhD

Published in the US in 2001, 2006
by DK Publishing, Inc.
375 Hudson Street
New York, New York 10014

DK books are available at special discounts for bulk
purchases for sales promotions, premiums, fund-
raising, or education use. For details, contact: DK
Publishing Special Markets, 375 Hudson Street, New
York, NY 10014 or SpecialSales@dk.com

A CIP catalog record for this book is available from
the Library of Congress.

ISBN 0-7566-2090-2

Reproduced by Colorscan, Singapore
Printed and bound by Star Standard, Singapore

see our complete catalog at
www.dk.com

special problems   **200**

An account of the dietary factors involved in some
children's disorders, with an explanation of how
superfoods can help.

food & disorders 201 ★ allergies 202
★ hyperactivity & ADHD 206 ★ eating
disorders 211

resources   **214**

A selection of organizations, societies, and Internet
sites that can help with many aspects of children's
eating and nutritional problems.

books to read   **216**

A list of useful books giving helpful information
and advice on various aspects of food for children,
including special diets.

index 217
acknowledgments 224

nutrition without numbers

"What's for supper, Mom?"

"A rich source of protein and energy, Children, with useful amounts of vitamin C, calcium, essential fatty acids, a little iodine, and some valuable B-complex vitamins."

In the real world, this answer does not add up to a delicious fish pie. But more and more, it is the way that nutritionists, dietitians, and self-appointed experts would have us think about our food.

Children do not eat fats, carbohydrates, vitamins, and minerals, they eat food. But the numbers approach is highly profitable for many food manufacturing companies. It allows them to add a few cheap nutrients to poor-quality food, and to persuade you that it is healthy for your children.

A canned "fruit drink," which is over 80 percent sugar, is described as containing "real fruit juice and vitamin C." A vanilla yogurt is said to be "made with all the valuable constituents of fresh milk and enriched with calcium, riboflavin, and vitamin B_{12}." You have to work out for yourself that it is 12½ percent pure sugar. A popular chocolate-flavored rice and corn breakfast cereal comes with "8 vitamins + iron" and is described as good "for maintaining healthy bones." Not so good for children's teeth, though: it is 38 percent sugar.

Claims to be "low fat" or"fat-free" are another instance of food manufacturers' sleight-of-hand. They have encouraged the public to believe that the greatest threat to health comes from over-consumption of fats, and equally, that it is fats that are chiefly responsible for today's hugely increased incidence of obesity. It's a belief that does not square with the facts. Between 1980 and 1991, consumption of fat in the US declined by nearly five percent, while the number of seriously overweight adults rose by nearly eight percent. It is sugar consumption that has rocketed: average daily intake is a staggering 35 teaspoons.

The same patterns of junk-food eating and little or no exercise are producing an epidemic of obesity in other countries, too. A horrifying study published in the *Lancet* in 1999 showed that at age six, 10 percent of British children were already obese, while by 15 the figure had risen to 17 percent. A study in Australia, found that nearly 10 percent of schoolchildren were obese and noted that a third of the family food budgets went for fast food.

what food slogans really mean

The term "low fat" can be misleading. "Low-fat" potato chips are still 21 percent fat. Yogurt is a low-fat food, anyway. All too often, the "low fat" claims are designed to distract you from all the other unhealthy things going into those potato chips, or that fruit-flavored yogurt devoid of fruit and crammed with sugar as well as lists of additives. "Sugar-free" or "light" is another useful term for food manufacturers. It means that sugar has been replaced by artificial sweeteners, the safety of which is open to question: see Danger Foods, pages 66–69.

The magic nutrition-by-numbers game is just as popular with the fast-food chains. It allows them to emphasize the one or two good nutrients in their products in order to distract attention from the horrendous amounts of fat, salt, and sugar with which they come packaged. It allows them virtually to suggest that the burger, French fries, and soft drink meal is a thoroughly healthy one for a growing child.

It is often claimed that children ate a healthier diet in the late 1930s and early '40s, despite rationing and shortages, than today's youngsters. This was not because mothers were specially knowledgeable about nutrition. Most may not have known that a broiled lamb chop supplies 28g of protein, 12g of fat, 2mgs of iron and 0.22mg of pyridoxine (vitamin B_6). What they did know was that a broiled lamb chop, a baked potato, and a helping of fresh green vegetables added up to nourishing and pleasurable food for their family.

problems in feeding today's children

It is not that we have lost the instinctive knowledge our grandparents possessed for knowing what is best for us and our children. Rather, we are living in a more complex and more stressful world.

Today's children, more often than not, have two working parents. Food shopping becomes a once-a-week trip to the local supermarket, often involving the whole family, when 7 days' eating is purchased in one trip, and shelf-life becomes a major criterion of excellence.

One of the fastest-growing sections of the modern supermarket is the range of ready-made meals from the cold foods section. These instant meals, which can keep for days in the refrigerator or be frozen for future use, can be a boon to the frantic home cook and a wonderful standby in emergencies. But they can never be a substitute, gastronomically or nutritionally, for food freshly prepared in your own home.

Outside the home, children have almost unfettered access to a huge range of unsuitable foods that parents can do little about. Children spend millions a year on snacks - potato chips and salty snacks, candy and carbonated drinks - on their way to and from school. And there are all those fast food hamburger chains where teenagers with plenty of pocket money like to gather with friends.

making home cooking easy

While today's parents have to make extra efforts at home to ensure that their children are regularly fed healthy and nutritious food, they are helped by today's greatly improved food-buying network. Local vegetable markets and supermarkets open early in the morning, and many stay open round the clock; there are farmers' markets, farm stands, and organic home delivery services. And of course there is the ever-expanding shopping mall of the Internet.

Even for busy working parents, it doesn't require all that much effort to stop on the way home and pick up chicken breasts and fresh vegetables for a stir-fry, or half a dozen eggs, fresh herbs, new potatoes, and salad-making ingredients for a summer evening omelette supper, or a chunk of Cheddar cheese and a good whole wheat loaf for Welsh rarebit. All these foods are superfoods. You will find them described in detail in this book, and there are recipes using them in many great, easy-to-make dishes.

The popular perception is that cooking is great to watch on TV but a chore to do in your own kitchen. It is certainly true that most of the recipes in this book will take longer to prepare than the time to unwrap a package and put a meal in the microwave.

But most of the recipes are for simple dishes that require little culinary skill to make, and a fairly short time to prepare. Your decision has to be whether these short moments of your leisure time are worth sacrificing in order to give your children the best chance of a long and healthy life.

Superfoods for Children takes you back to the old-fashioned principles of real home cooking that looks good, tastes good, and will definitely do your children good.

healthy eating need not cost a fortune

Serving healthy, nutritious meals for your family need not be any more expensive than feeding them a diet of French fries, hamburgers, potato chips, cookies, frozen pizzas, canned spaghetti, fried fish sticks and chicken nuggets, and cheap ice cream.

Even the seriously healthy stuff – the organic meat and poultry, eggs, fruit and vegetables, bread and rice – which once cost a lot more than ordinary fare is now generally less expensive than in the early days of its production.

Even if some manufactured food is cheaper, that doesn't make it a great value. And if you look at the enormous profits the food manufacturing giants make, and the astronomical sums they can afford to spend on advertising junk food, you might begin to wonder: are you really prepared to sacrifice your child's health to their profits?

Because their profits are based on using the very cheapest ingredients – refined white flour, white sugar, the cheapest margarines or vegetable oils,

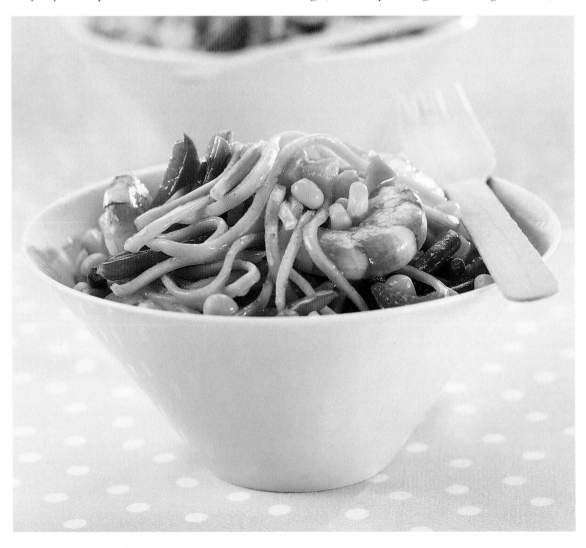

poor quality meat; on boosting their flavor or color with a few chemicals; and on giving them child-appeal with plenty of sugar and fat.

Buy one of those 6-packs of potato chips, for instance, and you'll be getting half a dozen less than 1oz/24g packages. They'll cost you 4–5 times the price of 1lb/500g potatoes at your greengrocer; and more than a third of their weight will be fat. They'll be very salty, too. And they certainly will not have been made from the best potatoes available on the market. For half the money, you could give your family wonderful new potatoes or crispy baked potatoes with delicious real butter.

You can take it for granted that the chicken in those chicken nuggets and the beef in frozen burgers will be from cut-price factory-farmed sources, that the flour in biscuits, cakes, pies will be the cheapest white, that the fish in those fingers may be little better than sludge, and that the 'fruit' drink may contain little more than 10 percent actual fruit. You can be sure, however, that at least two ingredients will be lavishly supplied in many of these foods - sugar and salt. And every shopper and cook knows how cheap those are.

cut down the costs

Most of the so-called "junk foods" do not actually form part of a proper meal anyway. They are the extras: the packages of potato chips and other snacks children buy on the way home from school, the ice creams and cookies brought to family outings, and the carbonated drinks which have replaced plain water in so many families: millions of children growing up today assume that a "drink" is something from a bottle or can, rather than a glassful of water from the tap.

Cut down on these extras and you'll have more money to spend on real food at mealtimes: your children won't have had their appetites ruined in advance, either.

Eating food when it's in season and locally grown is another way to slash the food bills. Out-of-season grapes and strawberries, green beans, and new potatoes imported from countries where its summer sooner than where you live, or hot all year round,

will always be more expensive than when they're in season. And jetlag won't enhance their nutritional value, either.

Unless yours is a vegetarian family, meat and fish will always be the biggest items in the weekly food bill. But it is only quite recently, and only in wealthy Western countries, that meat has come to form the centerpiece of the meal, with vegetables no more than accessories to the feast. Millions of people throughout the world live long, healthy and active lives on diets based mainly on grains and legumes, with just a little meat or fish for extra flavor. In China and in India, around the Mediterranean, and in Latin America, this is the normal way to eat, and wonderful food it is, too. Even when you're planning dishes which are based on meat, such as stews, casseroles, shepherds pie, or lasagna, you can always replace some of the meat with vegetables, and sometimes they can be substituted for it altogether.

Organic food *is* more expensive than conventionally-farmed produce. But the prices are beginning to come down as more and more farmers decide to grow organic crops. And as well as supermarkets, there are fast-growing numbers of farmers' markets where prices are much more competitive; there are local box schemes which are often excellent value; and there are organic retailers advertising on the internet. Shop around for the best bargains (see Resources, pages 214-15).

grow food at home

If you have a garden, even a small one, you can grow at least some of your own food organically. Grow arugula for salads, sorrel for soups, and plenty of spinach: all three grow fast and easily without too much attention.

Give the children a corner to grow their own food: they'll be much more likely to eat radishes, corn, or scallions that they've proudly produced themselves. Even if you only have a backyard, balcony or windowsill, use it to grow many of the herbs which contribute health as well as wonderful flavors to everyday eating: thyme, mint, chives, parsley, basil, oregano, rosemary.

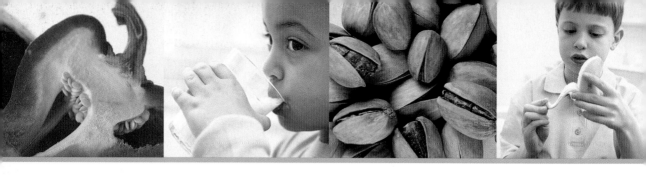

nutrition on a plate

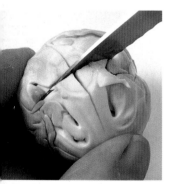

Small bodies need optimum nourishment to get them through their active days. The brains of children are even hungrier than their bodies, voracious in their need for oxygen, energy, and key nutrients. The foods that best supply these essential nutritional requirements are described here.

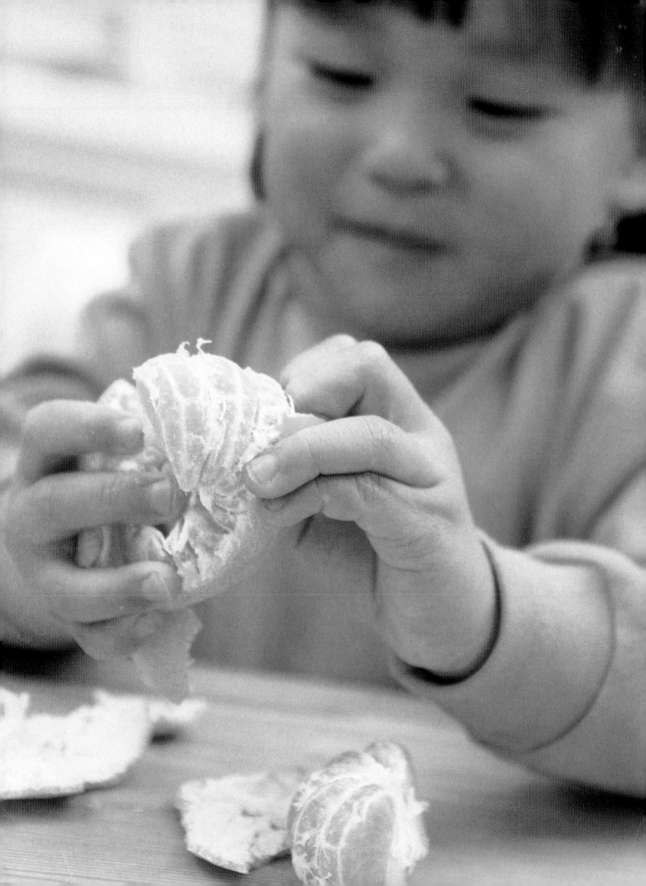

eating healthily

Follow the simple, practical guidelines illustrated by our plate for life and your family will get all the superfoods needed for health. The plate is divided into five sections, and, if you visualize it when you are shopping, planning the day's eating or thinking about the next meal, you'll never be far from eating healthily all the time.

A baby's first foods are necessarily few in number and must be carefully chosen. Once past babyhood, children benefit greatly from eating a wide range of foods, typified by the contents of our plate for life.

A third of the plate is filled with the vitality foods: all kinds of fruits, vegetables, or salads. Another third is filled with energy-giving foods: starchy carbohydrates including potatoes, pasta, whole wheat bread, brown rice, oats, and corn. The final third is divided into two larger segments and a much smaller segment.

One of the two larger segments is filled with the body-building foods, with lots of protein: lean meat, fish, poultry, eggs, beans, lentils, nuts, and seeds. The other is made up of body- and bone-building dairy products: milk, yogurt and cheeses.

The tiny segment is the place for fats, olive and other vegetable oils and treats such as butter, cream, sugar, chocolate, ice cream, and the white flour in croissants, French bread, pasta, and pizzas.

getting the balance right

The proportions of different types of food on this plate represent the ideal balance for healthy eating. Use these proportions as a guide, and you will always give your children enough starchy food for energy, enough protein for growth, enough fruit, vegetables, and salad for vitality, and enough calcium for strong bones, while keeping the amount of fats, oils, and dairy products within heart-healthy bounds. And there's still room for treats.

You'll only have to look at the meal you're putting in front of your children to know if you've got it right or wrong. A bowl of tomato soup with a crusty roll and a glass of milk; a homemade burger with oven-baked chips, peas and carrots; and fresh fruit salad with cream scores an A+ because there are plenty of the vitality foods, plenty of the energy foods, enough protein and body-building foods, and a little cream as a treat.

A cheeseburger and fries, with a milkshake, apple pie, and a carbonated drink, in contrast, rates only a C-. The meal provides adequate protein, but it also supplies masses of fat and salt, a huge amount of sugar, and just a leaf or two of tired lettuce and a little apple to represent the vitality foods.

You do not have to follow the proportions on the plate rigidly, or worry too much if the treats get out of hand from time to time: just try to stick to the general proportions. If your children are eating plenty of fruit and vegetables and the good energy foods, enough protein and enough body-building foods, and small amounts of healthy oils you can forget about adding up the numbers and percentages. Your children will be getting all the vitamins and minerals, trace elements and essential fatty acids, protein, carbohydrates and fats they need, and all the fiber as well.

A plate for life

Plan children's meals in the proportions of foods on this plate, and you will be sure they have a healthy diet.

• Vitality foods – fruits, vegetables, and salads – fill a third of the plate.

• Energy foods – starchy foods such as whole wheat bread, potatoes, pasta, brown rice, and oats – also fill a third of the plate.

• Body-building protein foods – lean meat, fish, eggs, legumes and nuts – fill 15 percent of the plate.

• Dairy foods, mainly milk products, also take up 15 per cent of the plate.

• Fats, including butter, cream, oils, and sugars; foods based on white flour; and "treats" should cover no more than 3 percent of the space on the plate.

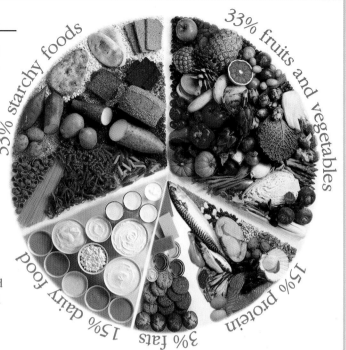

33% starchy foods

33% fruits and vegetables

15% protein

3% fats

15% dairy food

carbohydrates

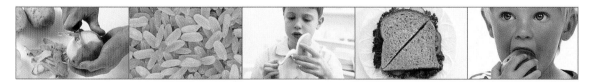

Carbohydrates are found in fruits; in grains such as wheat or rice; in legumes such as peas, beans, and lentils; in starchy vegetables like potatoes and carrots; in milk; and in sugar and honey. Carbohydrate foods are energy foods, and children need plenty of them, not only because they are naturally active and use up a lot of energy, but because they need energy for growth, too.

The best carbohydrate foods – whole wheat bread, brown rice, whole oats, beans, lentils, and fruit – supply more than just energy. They also contain important nutrients, and are rich in fiber to keep the digestive system functioning efficiently.

When these foods are refined or heavily processed, as are white bread and white rice, for instance, they lose not only large amounts of vital nutrients, but most of their fiber, too.

To take just the white flour that goes into our bread as an example: compared with whole wheat flour, white flour contains much less zinc, which children need to build resistance and to help with brain work; a great deal less magnesium, which is vital for the nervous system, and also for the absorption of calcium for the development of strong bones and teeth; and significantly less of the protein that is essential for body-building. Token amounts of major nutrients are added back when flour is baked into bread, but not for other uses. Much the same losses occur when rice and grains are refined. And the white sugar produced when sugar beet and sugar cane are processed has absolutely no nutritional value at all, except for a lot of energy-giving calories which have been styled "empty" for this reason. Brown sugar and honey at least contain traces of some key nutrients.

carbohydrates and glucose

There is another downside to highly refined carbohydrate foods. When they are eaten, the sugars they contain are broken down into glucose during the process of digestion. Glucose, or blood sugar as it is also called, is the fuel our bodies run on. The glucose circulating in our bloodstream after a carbohydrate meal is transferred to cells for instant use, and any surplus is converted into glycogen and stored as fuel in the liver, ready to be "switched on" for use whenever it is needed. The hormone insulin, which is secreted by the pancreas, is responsible for this storage job.

Eat a slice of whole wheat bread, a bowl of lentils, or a few ripe apricots and the sugars in them are broken down into glucose quite slowly. But eat a couple of cookies, a bowl of cornflakes, or a chocolate bar, all of which are known as "high-glycemic" foods because they are rapidly absorbed, and the sugars they contain will be broken down very quickly into glucose, sending the level in the bloodstream soaring.

The pancreas responds to this abnormal situation by pumping out extra insulin, and blood-sugar levels drop sharply. You are now suffering – if only in passing – from hypoglycemia or low blood sugar, sometimes called the "Sugar Blues." Children who eat a plateful of sugary cereals for breakfast may experience this dive in blood sugar a couple of hours later, making them jittery, unable to concentrate, and craving a little sugary fix.

These fluctuations in blood-sugar levels have been linked to a wide range of health problems. Long-term, they can be responsible for high blood pressure, obesity, diabetes, and heart disease in adults. In children, they may be responsible for disruptive behavior, hyperactivity and an inability to concentrate. One of the most common symptoms of low blood sugar is fatigue – which may account for the state of permanent exhaustion in which so many of today's teenagers appear to live.

Researchers have discovered another consequence of the constant insulin "highs" produced by yoyo-ing blood sugar levels. Insulin stimulates an enzyme called lipoprotein-lipase, which directs circulating fatty acids into fat-cell storage, thus increasing body weight, instead of into ordinary cells to be burned up by their power-plants, the mitochondria. Children who are constantly snacking on cookies, potato chips, cakes, ice cream, and candy bars will tend to put on weight – and obesity among children is a growing problem.

vary the carbohydrates

Give children whole wheat bread, brown rice, and nourishing cooked oatmeal most of the time, and save the sweet rolls, cookies, and pizzas, for treats. The more nourishing foods are more filling and satisfying, too, so children will not keep asking for odd snacks. There's no need to ban sugar, but choose unrefined cane sugar instead of white, and be very stingy with it. Honey can often replace sugar, though it should not be given to babies under one year since, in rare cases, bacteria found in honey can cause botulism.

It is a good idea to vary the carbohydrates in your children's meals. Most modern Western diets over-emphasize a few basic foodstuffs – wheat-based ones in particular. Toast for breakfast, bread in some form in the middle of the day, cakes and cookies after school, and pasta or pizza for supper add up to an awful lot of just one food. Growing numbers of children are sensitive to certain foods, which can give them severe digestive and other problems. Top of the list of these problem foods is wheat, closely followed by dairy foods, and the orange juice which is most babies' first drink after milk. (See Special Problems, pages 200–213, for advice on recognizing the potential problem foods and how to deal with them.)

protein

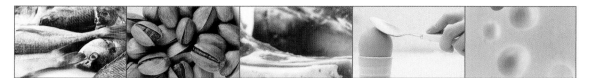

Protein is found in a wide variety of foods including anything made from cereals such as wheat and oats; in rice, eggs, cheese, fish, poultry, meat, nuts, and seeds; and in all varieties of beans, peas, and lentils. Generally speaking, protein derived from animal sources is a complete protein on its own, whereas, with the exception of soy beans, you need to combine cereals with legumes to obtain complete protein from vegetable sources. This is commonly seen in ethnic foods like rice and black-eyed peas in the West Indies, or chapattis with dal in India.

Protein is essential for the building of every single one of the body's cells and it is constantly being used and replaced. Because babies, children, and teenagers are growing rapidly they tend to need more protein in relation to their weight than adults. Pregnant women also need extra protein for the creation of new cells in their growing babies.

In the developed countries, adult protein deficiency is extremely unusual, except for those suffering from eating disorders. But it's less rare to find children whose protein intake is marginal or low, since children are more inclined to eat a limited range of foods and to develop passing obsessions with particular foods eaten to the exclusion of others. But don't be too alarmed if your child will only eat baked beans, potato chips or French fries. 100 grams of each provides 15, 5.1, and 6.3 grams of protein respectively.

Children's need for protein varies with age, and boys and girls have the same daily requirements up to the age of 10. After that age their requirements differ, as the chart, right, indicates. However, this does not denote the amount of protein-containing foods that children need to eat, because no food is made up of just protein. Vegetables contain 5 percent or less protein, and fruits contain very little. Eggs, cheese, fish, meat and poultry, peanuts, beans, lentils, cereals, and bread contain between 10 and 30 percent protein and usually provide over 80 percent of a child's daily protein consumption.

The following list of foods, showing the amount of protein in an average portion, will give you an idea of how much protein your children are obtaining from the food they eat:

- 3½oz/100g white fish have 18 grams of protein
- 1¼ cups/300ml whole milk have 10 grams
- two boiled eggs have 14 grams
- 7oz/200g baked beans have 8 grams
- one slice of wholemeal bread has 3 grams
- 2oz/60g of peanuts have 14 grams
- a 1 inch/2½cm cube of Cheddar has 12 grams
- an average hamburger has 10 grams
- one fish stick has 4 grams.

Freezing does not much alter the amount of protein present in foods, although cooking can make some difference. Slightly cooked proteins are thought to be more easily digested than raw; if you overcook red meat until it is tough, the protein will be less available because the digestive juices will have trouble breaking it down.

Daily protein requirements of children

Age group	Boys	Girls
0–3 months	12.5g	12.5g
7–9 months	13.7g	13.7g
10–12 months	14.9g	14.9g
4–6 years	19.7g	19.7g
7–10 years	28.3g	28.3g
11–14 years	42.0g	41.2g
15–18 years	55.2g	45.0g

The body is not able to store protein, and if excessive amounts are eaten they will be converted into sugars and fats. The idea that feeding your child lots of protein instead of starchy foods will be less fattening is wrong and may well be more harmful to health. It is particularly important not to feed too much protein food to small babies (up to the age of 9–12 months). Their immature kidneys cannot deal with the breakdown products that build up in the bloodstream, and this can lead to serious problems.

It is perfectly possible to raise your child as a vegetarian and still ensure he receives adequate amounts of protein. You will need to pay particular attention to maintaining iron and vitamin B_{12} intake, but there is no problem with providing sufficient vegetable-based protein to ensure normal growth (see Vegetarian Children, pages 104–7).

fats

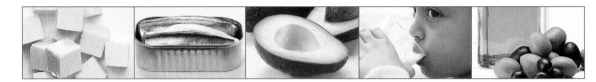

Science has now established an irrefutable link between heart disease and breast cancer and a high intake of animal fat in the diet. Many Western governments have responded by aiming to reduce the total percentage of calories their populations obtain from fat in their diet. In the US the figure is 30 percent, the equivalent of 70 or 75 grams of fat in an adult's approximately 2000 calorie daily diet, which seems to be the level above which heart disease and breast cancer become more prevalent.

As there is growing evidence that the seeds of heart disease are sown in childhood, possibly even in the womb, it is clearly never too early to teach your children eating habits that control their intake of total fats and particularly of saturated fats.

Saturated, polyunsaturated, monounsaturated, trans-fats, cholesterol, omega-3, omega-6 – all fats, all confusing, but are they good or bad? Do children need any of them in their daily diet? The answer to the last question is that they most certainly do: growing children need to derive quite a high percentage of their energy intake from fat – 50 percent up to the age of one year, and 35 percent thereafter. Some fats are essential to enable the body to absorb the fat-soluble vitamins A, D, E, and K. The essential point is to understand what kinds of fat there are and how much children need.

Saturated fats are nearly all animal fats: butter, lard, the fat in meat, and the fat in cheese, cream, and milk. Some vegetables also produce saturated fat, especially coconut and palm. The body is able to manufacture its own saturated fatty acids so you do not need to eat them.

Polyunsaturated fats are found mainly in vegetable oils like soy bean, corn, sunflower, and safflower. They also occur in oily fish. They are extremely important and should form a regular part of every child's diet.

Monounsaturated fats occur mostly in olive oil, nuts, and seeds and canola oil, and are important as heart protectors.

Essential fatty acids include the omega-6 and omega-3 fatty acids that are vital building blocks of body cells, especially brain and central-nervous-system tissue. Without them, normal development of the baby's brain during pregnancy and in early childhood can be adversely affected.

Recent studies have indicated a lack of some of these essential fatty acids in the diets of pregnant vegetarian women. The omega-6 fats are found in safflower, soy and sunflower oil, and the omega-3s are abundant in oily fish and in soy bean, canola and walnut oils.

Cholesterol
It is generally accepted that levels of cholesterol in the blood are a key indication of an individual's risk of heart disease. But cholesterol is an essential constituent of every cell in the body. Happily, the liver makes all that you need so there is no requirement to get it from food.

Trans-fats,
found mostly in margarines, are the real villains. Good natural foods are always preferable to anything manufactured in a factory and margarine is the prime example. Trans-fats are even more dangerous for your child's heart than saturated fats, so small amounts of unsalted butter are undeniably better than any margarine.

keeping a watch on calories
Calorie content is a main reason for being very careful with a child's fat intake. Of all the components of our food, fat contains the highest number of calories by weight and, with the exception of fat-reduced spreads, all fats –

whether saturated, unsaturated or essential fatty acids – will give very nearly the same number of calories in every ½ cup/100g (more than twice as many as starchy foods). Three ounces/one hundred grams of boiled new potatoes contain only 76 calories. But turn the potatoes into French fries with added fat and the potatoes will amount to 253 calories.

We get 50 percent of our daily fat intake from meat, milk, cream, cheese, eggs, and oily fish; 30 percent from butter, margarine, and other fats and oils; and 8 percent from food items such as cookies, cakes, and pastries.

The first step towards ensuring children do not get more fat than they need is to cut down on all the visible fats (i.e., the ones you can see): butter, cheese, cream, the fat around steak or chops, or on the outside of a slice of ham or bacon. Much more difficult is to avoid the hidden fats in meat products like luncheon meats, pies and pastries, cookies, cakes, Danish pastry, and chocolate. These are insidious and the only way to control them in your child's diet is to read all labels very carefully – only occasionally buying high-fat foods and in small quantities.

The chart below shows just how little of some of these high-fat foods your child needs to eat to provide 10 grams of fat – almost a third of his total recommended consumption for a day.

Fat in foods
The fat content of some foods, eaten in quantity by children, is alarmingly high. The table below lists popular foods and their fat content. A 35g piece of quiche, for example, contains 10g of fat.

Food amount containing **10g** (⅓oz) of fat

Food	Amount	Food	Amount	Food	Amount
Chocolate cookies	35g	Lamb chop with fat	30g	Cream cheese	20g
Shortbread cookies	40g	Average meat patty	50g	Processed cheese	25g
Sponge cake	40g	Fried shrimp	55g	Cheddar cheese	30g
Cheesecake	30g	Butter, Margarine	12g	Quiche	35g
Fried bacon	20g	Lard, Vegetable oil	10g	Potato chips	30g
Fried chicken w/skin	25g	Heavy cream	20g	French fries (frozen)	50g
Pizza w/cheese	35g	Light cream	50g	Milk chocolate	35g
Pork sausage	30g	Mayonnaise	12g		

minerals

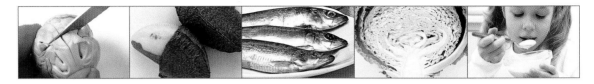

Because of modern intensive-farming methods, soil that has been artificially fertilized and had the same crop grown on it for years may have had its natural stores of minerals depleted. The crops and the animals fed on them may then contain less than we need, and that can be a health hazard for children.

Minerals and trace elements are of special interest to us, since deficiencies are often overlooked as the cause of illness. From birth onwards they are essential for growth, development, natural resistance, and all-round health. Make sure your family gets plenty of minerals by eating all the foods listed here – ideally, organically grown.

Zinc is vital for growth, healthy sex organs, insulin production, and natural resistance. Lack of zinc can lead to weight loss, skin diseases, ulcers and acne, loss of taste and smell, and brittle nails.

People with anorexia nervosa have very low levels of zinc; ask your child's physician if a zinc supplement might help.

A lack of zinc may be linked to ADHD (see page 206), and could even start before birth if the mother is low on her own intake. Zinc, in food or as a supplement, helps with teenage acne.

Best zinc sources are shellfish (especially oysters), lamb, liver, steak, garlic, Brazil nuts, pumpkin seeds, eggs, sardines, oats, crab, almonds, and chicken.

Selenium is a key factor in the immune system. It is also important for giving protection against heart disease, skin problems, and increased risk of cancer.

In some Western countries, selenium intake has dropped markedly in recent years. This is all the more alarming in view of the fact that current research shows that normally harmless viruses can become dangerously virulent when living in a body that is deficient in selenium.

This may all seem far removed from your baby or child, but making sure the diet is full of selenium-rich foods is not only protection now but will help protect health throughout the child's life.

Best sources are whole wheat bread made from Canadian and North American flour, Brazil nuts, butter, oily fish, liver, and kidney.

Magnesium is essential in many of the body's enzyme functions, and helps maintain a balanced distribution of calcium, potassium, and sodium in individual cells. It is vital for growth and also as part of the cell-repair mechanism. It is, in addition, one of the minerals that enables nerve pulses to be transmitted from cell to cell.

Magnesium deficiency can be the result of bad eating habits, malnutrition, anorexia nervosa, inability to eat because of mouth or tooth problems, or poor absorption due to digestive disease. Eating too much uncooked bran increases magnesium loss from the body, as can excessive consumption of fats, vitamin D, and calcium. Some prescribed drugs, including some antibiotics and diuretics, can increase magnesium loss, too.

A magnesium deficiency can cause hyperactivity, apathy, exhaustion, fatigue, cramps, tremors, insomnia, palpitations, and low blood-sugar levels. This vital mineral is also required by the body to aid good calcium absorption (see opposite).

The best food sources of magnesium are soy beans, nuts, whole wheat flour, brown rice, dried fruit, and bananas. All green vegetables are also very good sources of this mineral.

Iron is the substrate in hemoglobin to which oxygen binds, providing the red coloring of the blood. This hemoglobin transports the oxygen from the air we breathe to every cell of the body. Iron helps keep children cheerful and active. Without enough, your child is vulnerable to anemia, fatigue, depression, and palpitations, and will look pale.

Kelp (seaweed), molasses, pig's liver, beef, black pudding, oily fish like salmon, herring, and sardines, shellfish, kidney beans, Brazil nuts, dates, raisins, lentils, chickpeas, peanuts, chicken, egg yolk, soy beans, and peas are good sources of iron. A reasonable-sized portion of liver, chili con carne, or a home-cooked burger or steak, with green vegetables, peas or beans, provides the daily need. Contrary to popular belief, spinach is not the best source of iron, since it also contains oxalic acid, which makes it more difficult for the body to absorb.

Copper works with iron to make red blood corpuscles, important for bone formation, breakdown of cholesterol and the skin pigment melanin. Deficiency can lead to anemia, hair problems, high cholesterol and dry skin.

Children who eat nuts, beef, liver, lamb, butter, barley, and olive oil get all the copper they need.

Calcium is a vital mineral for the formation and continuing strength of bones and teeth, and is particularly important during pregnancy, breast-feeding, childhood, and in the teenage years. In later life, both women and men are at risk of osteoporosis (brittle-bone disease), which is caused partly by a combination of too little calcium in the diet and poor absorption, and partly by the fact that bones naturally lose density as we get older.

The time to do something positive about protecting bones for life is in childhood. A diet which contains lots of calcium-rich foods is the first step. And children should be encouraged to be active, participate in sports, and get plenty of fresh air and sunshine, which makes vitamin D (another substance, like magnesium, that is needed for good calcium absorption).

Milk, yogurt and cheese are great sources of calcium, so encourage a taste for them in your children and make them part of their regular daily food. Canned sardines with the bones included, lots of greens, and dried fruit, nuts, beans, and good bread are other good food sources of calcium. Eating plenty of them will guarantee your children grow up with strong bones and teeth.

Iodine is essential for the proper working of the thyroid gland, which produces hormones that control many of the body's functions. It also gives some degree of protection against radiation damage to the thyroid. Lack of iodine will cause lethargy, skin thickening, hair loss, growth problems, and goiter (thyroid enlargement). Too much, on the other hand, may cause overactivity of the thyroid.

Seaweed and sea fish are the only dependable sources of iodine. But beware of taking too much of the kelp (seaweed) supplements, which can be high in iodine – few of them are standardized – and may cause thyroid problems.

Manganese is needed for the formation of a number of enzymes, bone formation, muscle action, and fertility. A lack of it may cause bone and disc problems and high blood-sugar levels. It is found in all wholegrain cereals, nuts, and tea – one cup of tea provides nearly half the daily requirement.

Potassium is essential for the proper functioning of all the human body's cells and nervous tissue. It is present in all foods except oils, fats, and sugars: bananas are a great source. It can be dissolved in the cooking water of vegetables, so save the vegetable cooking water for soups, gravy, and stews.

vitamins & antioxidants

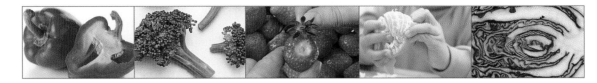

Antioxidants have been the great nutritional revelation of the past decade or so. They are powerfully protective plant chemicals found in the bright pigments of fruits and vegetables, and form the body's best defence against attack by unfriendly molecules called free radicals, which are generated both in our bodies and environmentally by pollutants such as pesticides, tobacco smoke, and stress. Free-radical damage has been linked to cancer, heart disease, wrinkles, cataracts, and more.

The earliest known antioxidants were vitamins C and E, and beta-carotene, which is turned in the body into vitamin A. It is now known that the pigments which give fruits and vegetables their glowing colors are rich in these wonderful protective factors – so children should feast on brilliantly colored seasonal fruits and vegetables.

Although health departments the world over are concerned to keep everyone informed about how many vitamins and minerals we should all be taking every day – given as RDA ("recommended daily allowance") figures on many food labels – they make no allowance for the huge variations in the actual nutrient content of today's foods. Intensive growing methods, transporting, storage, freshness, and handling can all reduce the level of vitamins and antioxidants in foods. And that's before you buy them, take them home, and cook them. The theoretical vitamin content of what ends up on your child's plate is often a great deal more than the reality of what is eaten.

There is also an enormous difference between what children need to avoid deficiency diseases, and the amounts needed to keep them in good health and to protect them against serious illness.

The following list describes in detail what the vitamins do and how much you theoretically have to eat to achieve the RDAs. Obviously, children's requirements vary with age, but from about 11 years old their needs are much the same as the adult quantities that are specified here.

Vitamin A is essential for growth, for the skin, and for night and color vision. Get all you need for a day from: *2oz/60g liver; 1½oz/45g mature carrots; 2½oz/75g spinach, butter or margarine; or 4oz/125g broccoli with 2oz/60g Cheddar cheese in a sauce.*

Vitamin C prevents scurvy, aids wound-healing and iron absorption, and is a vital and protective antioxidant. The daily dose is in: *2 teaspoons raisins, half a green bell pepper, a lemon, an orange, half a large grapefruit, a kiwifruit, or 3oz/90g raw red cabbage.*

Vitamin D contributes to the system of calcium absorption, essential for bone formation. Lack of vitamin D causes rickets in children and bone disorders in adults. The action of sunlight on the skin produces vitamin D, so encourage lots of outdoor activities. Some cultures are more often at risk for vitamin-D deficiency as a result of their their traditional diet and lifestyle, which includes wearing clothes that expose very little skin to the sun.

The 10µg that is essential will be obtained from: *1 teaspoon cod-liver oil, 1½oz/45g herring, 2oz/60g mackerel, 2½ oz/75g canned salmon or tuna, or 4½oz/140g canned sardines. Eggs also contain the vitamin.*

Vitamin B$_1$, Thiamine's main function is during the conversion of carbohydrates into energy. If you live on a high-starch diet, as some vegetarians do, the need for vitamin B$_1$ increases. Your daily dose can be had from: *2oz/60g cod roe, 2½oz/75g wheatgerm, 3½oz/100g Brazil nuts or peanuts. Oatmeal, bacon, pork, organ meats, and bread are all good sources, too.*

Vitamin B$_2$, Riboflavin, is vital for growth and for the skin and mucous membranes. *6 eggs, 1 quart/900ml milk, 2oz (60g) liver or kidney, or 8oz/250g Cheddar cheese will each supply the 1.3g you need. Beef, mackerel, almonds, cereals, and poultry are also good sources.*

Vitamin B$_6$, Pyridoxine, helps to release energy from protein. It is essential for growth and the functioning of the immune and nervous systems. It may also overcome some of the side-effects of the contraceptive pill. *Fish, meat, liver, and cheese are good sources. A large banana and half an avocado will provide the daily dose. A portion of cod, salmon, or a broiled herring will give you nearly all you need.*

Folic acid is vital during a child's growth and development as well as during pregnancy, and deficiency is linked to birth defects such as spina bifida. Also vital throughout life for protection against heart disease. *The best sources are dark green vegetables, liver, kidney, nuts, whole wheat bread and wholegrain cereals. An average portion of lamb's liver supplies 250μg, spinach 140μg and kidney beans, frozen peas, chickpeas, and raw red cabbage all around 75μg of the essential 200μg.*

children and vitamin supplements

The burning question most people ask about vitamins and their children is, "Do my children need to take extra vitamins?" The theoretical answer is "No, not if you are all eating a well-balanced diet, and using a wide variety of foods."

In fact, few people manage to do this, and even fewer persuade their partners or children to do it. Pressures of time, working parents, and the relentless force of the fast-food industry all make it more difficult.

Buying vitamin supplements can be very confusing. Do you choose a multivitamin; six individual vitamins (and if so, which ones?); mega-dose, slow-release, or vegetarian capsules; tablets made without gluten, yeast, colorings or sugars; a brand with 70 different ingredients, or one with five?

You may also waste money on supplements your children don't need, and which may do more harm than good. Single vitamins and minerals certainly have a place but, as a general rule, they – and certainly, the high-dose ones – should be taken on the advice of a doctor or nutritionist.

If you are giving vitamin supplements to children, make sure that you only buy those specifically formulated for the age of your child and that you do not exceed the stated dose. While current government guidelines recommend that all children under the age of 5 should take a supplement of vitamins A, C, and D, as a general rule of thumb, most children should not need anything more than a simple multivitamin and mineral, unless they have some underlying health problem or are on a very unusual diet. In these circumstances, get professional advice before you start dosing your children.

Note:
'μg' in some of the quantities mentioned here indicates micrograms; one microgram is equivalent to one millionth of a gram.

organic foods

Organic produce is taking an increasingly prominent place in our thinking about food standards. It is **grown** without the **many chemicals** of conventional foods, generally **tastes** better, and contains more nutrients, too. It is certainly the **kind of food** we want our children to eat.

Remember that a baby's central nervous system is developing but immature, and that it's immune system is still, like the baby, in its infancy. There has been little research into the effects on very small children of the multiple chemical cocktail that goes into much food production. Some leading allergy experts maintain that it is not atmospheric pollution that produces problems such as the ever-increasing incidence of asthma among our children so much as the damage to their immune systems from chemicals and additives in food. It seems only sensible to use as much organic produce in babies' diets as possible to remove one major factor that could potentially be damaging. The same remains true as your baby grows into a toddler, school child, teenage, and adolescent.

There are many reasons for trying to bring children up as organically as possible – which is much easier to do than it once was, with an increasing number of organic food sources, from farm stands to mail order Internet sites, and with many supermarkets greatly extending their range of organic foods, both fresh and processed.

avoiding additives

One important reason for going organic is to avoid the huge list of artificial additives that find their way into commercially produced and processed foods, from artificial sweeteners to coloring agents.

Many of the orange drinks that four- and five-year-olds drink so avidly contain very little of the citrus fruit and a great many additives. Avoid all the chemicals and added sugar by giving children pure organic fruit juices diluted 50/50 with water – if they like them fizzy, use mineral water. Look out, too, for the organic juices without added sugar, other sweeteners or agrochemical residues that major manufacturers are now producing.

An even more important reason for going organic centers on the question of nutritional value. Without a doubt, organically produced crops are higher in nutrients than their conventionally-grown counterparts. Studies consistently show higher contents of vitamins A and C in organically-grown fruits and vegetables, for instance. The organic farmer uses traditional methods of crop rotation, green manure planting, composting and organic fertilizing to keep the soil in good condition and to replace nutrients taken up by previous crops.

Intensive commercial cultivation relies on artificial fertilizers which replace only the nutrients essential to grow the crops, with scant regard for their nutritional quality. Intensive livestock producers have to use feed supplemented with minerals and vitamins to replace those missing from their own feed crops, and non-organic produce has a much higher water content and contains less of these essential vitamins and minerals.

Other things besides nutrients may be missing or have a reduced presence, in intensively-raised livestock. Professor Mike Parizza, studying cattle meat at the University of Wisconsin, isolated a special fat called conjugated linoleic acid (CLA), a powerful anti-carcinogen. This essential fatty acid proved to be a key factor in weight control: the more CLA in the diet the more the body stores surplus calories as muscle rather than fat. Professor Parizza's research also showed that the highest levels of CLA were found in beef raised naturally on grass.

It's extraordinary that in all the food legislation there are laws that cover everything from seeds to packaging, from storage to handling, from dairy hygiene to clean food shops, even down to the size and shape of bananas, and from sell-by dates to labeling. But there is no law that makes testing for nutritional quality obligatory.

organic foods taste great

And a final reason for going organic: most organically-grown foods have full, rich flavors, and superb textures – particularly important where children are concerned.

Take a bite out of an organic then a commercially grown apple; dip your organically grown stoneground flour whole wheat bread toast into the yolk of an organic free-range egg and compare it to a slice of white sliced commercial bread in the pale anemic yolk of a non-organic egg; savor an organic freshly harvested new potato with any non-organic variety you care to name; you won't need a degree in food technology to tell the difference – and neither will your children.

Organic food is best for all these reasons, and it does not really matter whether you choose it for taste, safety, or to protect the environment, and it does not matter whether or not you can switch to a totally organic diet, since every organic product you consume is better for your health and better for the planet, too.

Try beginning with organically-grown versions of those foods where the risk of chemical residues are high – root vegetables such as carrots, or lettuces and other salad greens, for instance – or where farm production has been called seriously into question, such as with beef, or, if you have a young baby, with organic formula milk. Such foods can do nothing but good for growing children.

If you're pregnant or have plans to become so, if you are responsible for the diets of young children, or if you are suffering or recovering from serious illness, it is really important that you make organic food as big a part of your regular food consumption as you can possibly afford.

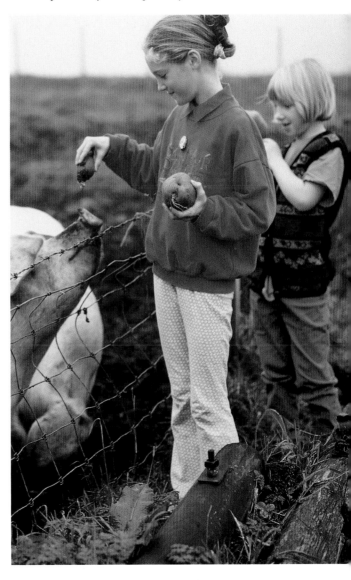

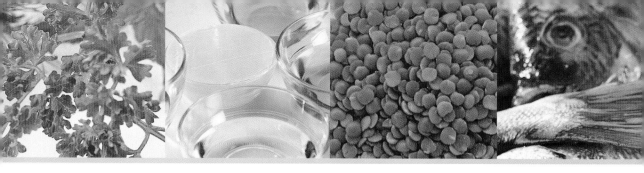

superfoods

Here are over 130 foods – vegetables,
fruits, dairy products, grains, nuts and seeds,
meats, fish, herbs, and oils – that provide
the building blocks for the irresistible

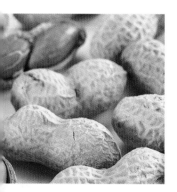

recipes and menu plans in
Superfoods for Children. Use the
foods to build the kind of diet
your children need for healthy

growth – and which they'll also enjoy eating.

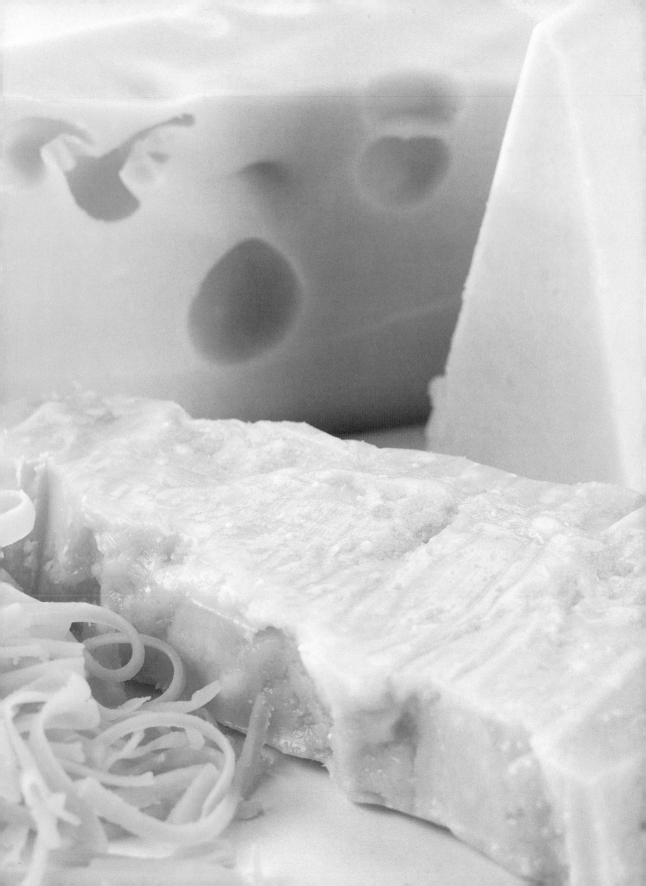

super vegetables

Green is nature's favorite color, and green leafy vegetables are the cornerstone of healthy eating, reducing cancer rates and heart disease and increasing longevity. Feast your family on these vital greens, on earthy roots, and on the many other rainbow-hued members of the vegetable kingdom.

cabbage

Cabbage has for centuries been valued for its healing properties and as a stress-buster. Today, researchers are finding that cabbage also has enormous cancer-prevention value. Studies have shown that in areas where people eat large quantities of cabbage and its close relatives, including the superfoods cauliflower and broccoli, some cancers, such as cancer of the lung, colon, breast, and uterus, are far less common.

This anti-cancer effect is attributed to phyto-chemicals (protective plant chemicals), especially glucosinolates, found in all the brassicas. As soon as the leaves are chopped, crushed, juiced, or cooked, enzymes are released which convert the glucosinolates into indoles, a group of chemicals that is anti-carcinogenic. Studies with animals have shown that cabbage can have a mild protective effect against radiation, and this may work for people, too, especially if the cabbage is eaten raw.

Cabbage contains healing mucilaginous substances similar to those produced by the mucous membrane of the gut and stomach for their own protection. It is also rich in sulfur, a mineral often in short supply in our diets but vital to healthy skin and joints. It is valuable for chest infections and is a powerful antibacterial.

QUICK FOOD IDEA

Add both the cooking water and the leftover shreds of cooked cabbage to a quickly prepared vegetable soup for a satisfyingly meaty flavor.

Cabbage, like the other brassicas, becomes indigestible if overcooked and loses much of its healing power. Wash it well and shred it, then cook it in a tightly lidded pan over a low heat in a tablespoon or so of water for 2–3 minutes only. When it's done, add a teaspoon of butter and a dusting of nutmeg, or a spoonful of oil and lemon juice. Or stir-fry it, or eat it raw in Coleslaw, a salad that many children love (see page 198).

A **rich source** of folic acid, sulfur, vitamin C, beta-carotene, and fiber.

broccoli

Another brassica, with the same cancer-fighting properties as cabbage. Serve broccoli raw in florets with a dip (see page 149) or steamed for 2–3 minutes until just tender. Stir-frying is another excellent way to cook broccoli and the other brassicas to enjoy them at their health-giving best.

A **rich source** of potassium and beta-carotene, and a **good source** of iron; the latter is well-absorbed by the body, because broccoli contains vitamin C, which is essential for this process.

cauliflower

Although cauliflower contains the same cancer-fighting compounds as other brassicas, it is less rich in beta-carotene, riboflavin, and folic acid, all of which are easily destroyed by over-cooking. Cauliflower is a great crunchy dipping vegetable.

If you do cook it, be sure to add some of its tender young inner leaves for extra vitamin C and beta-carotene.

Interestingly, there is more available beta-carotene in cooked brassica vegetables than in raw.

asparagus

Children love finger-food, and dipping asparagus spears in a little melted butter or mayonnaise is a messy treat. Asparagus is a good resistance-booster because it has huge amounts of beta-carotene, which is also essential for the development of healthy skin and lungs. There is an added bonus of significant amounts of antioxidant and protective vitamin E. Cook and serve asparagus soon after you buy it, as it spoils when stored too long.

QUICK FOOD IDEA

Use stem trimmings and cooking water, plus herbs and seasoning, for a quickly made soup.

A **rich source** of beta-carotene, vitamin E, and folic acid, asparagus is also a **good source** of minerals and of fiber.

turnips

Not every child's favorite vegetable, but well worth including in winter soups, casseroles or roasted vegetables, because of their high sulfur content which will help protect young lungs from infection. An old country cure for coughs was made by hollowing out a raw turnip, filling it with brown sugar and giving children teaspoon-size doses of the runny liquid which formed.

A **useful source** of fiber, calcium, phosphorus, potassium and some B vitamins.

carrots

Tiny young carrots taste delicious but contain far fewer vital carotenoids than the much darker-colored mature carrots, which contain so much beta-carotene that just one average-size carrot provides enough beta-carotene for a whole day's requirement.

Beta-carotene is converted in the body to vitamin A, vital for healthy skin and mucous membranes and, therefore, for the lungs and the entire respiratory system. Vitamin A is also essential for good night vision.

It is now well-established that eating generous quantities of carrots provides increased protection against the risks of some cancers, especially those of the lungs and breast.

Carrots have also long been used in the treatment of diarrhea, particularly among small children and infants for whom carrot purée is both healthy food and good medicine. Scrape 1lb/500g

QUICK FOOD IDEA

Put carrot sticks on the table for children to nibble at while they wait for you to dish up. Serve them with dips (see page 149) or grated in a creamy dressing as part of a crudités starter.

dark orange carrots, boil in enough water to cover until very soft, press through a food mill, and add boiled water to bring the amount up to 4 cups/1 liter. Refrigerate for up to 24 hours; feed the liquid to a baby by bottle and the solids by the spoonful.

If possible, buy organic. Carrots readily accumulate alarming levels of pesticide residues – so much so that it's good advice is to top, tail, and scrape them before eating.

A **good source** of beta-carotene, and **contain** reasonable amounts of vitamins C and E.

potatoes

Potatoes are very good for your children. They are not fattening, but filling, full of energy, and rich in a number of good nutrients, including enough vitamin C to keep scurvy at bay even in winter. Obviously, serving children French fries every day is not a good idea, but boiled or baked potatoes contain only 100 calories per 3½oz/100 grams, and you can serve them with baked beans, salad, a poached egg, cottage cheese, cold chicken, garlic mayonnaise, or spicy chili to make an inexpensive and ribsticking meal.

It's worth noting that thin, French fries are much more unhealthy than old-fashioned fat potato wedges. The fries absorb far more fat and are covered in salt, both of which are best avoided in any quantity.

Potatoes are a **good source** of vitamin C, fiber, some potassium, folic acid, iron, and protein.

QUICK FOOD IDEAS

Potatoes Juventus: peel potatoes and cut into ½in/1cm cubes. Put in a baking dish with 2 tbsp olive oil, tossing to coat them. Add a couple of sprigs of rosemary and bake until golden and tender.

For healthy mashed potato use olive oil, not butter.

Pairing potatoes with cabbage is a good way to persuade children to eat greens: try Bubble and Squeak (page 174) and Colcannon (page 141).

Sweet potatoes are a tuber, not related to potatoes, but they are so rich in beta-carotene they belong in any healthy diet. Cut them in fat wedges and oven roast; cook them with ordinary potatoes and mash together; add them to soups, casseroles, or stews.

spinach

Its iron content is not the best reason for eating spinach – sorry Popeye. It is, however, a very rich source of the dark green plant "blood," chlorophyll, so is valuable both in preventing and treating anemia. Children may not relish platefuls of spinach, but tender, young leaves in a salad with crispy bacon and slices of avocado may tempt them.

Spinach contains high levels of two carotenoids, lutein and xeaxanthin, which protect not only against cancer, but more particularly against a major cause of poor sight in later years called age-related macular degeneration. People who eat spinach and other dark green vegetables on a regular basis are less than half as likely as those who do not to develop this disease. It's never too soon to start protecting eyesight.

A **rich source** of the carotenoids, and a **good source** of potassium, vitamin E, and folic acid.

onions, leeks, garlic

Onions, garlic, leeks, scallions, chives, and shallots all belong to the same family, the alliums. You might think that these strongly-flavored vegetables lack child-appeal, but in fact most children love them as onion rings with their hamburgers, as garlic bread in the pizzeria, or made into a hearty onion soup on a cold winter's day.

As well as that great taste, onions and garlic are a family medicine chest in themselves. As intensive modern research has shown, they protect the lungs, the heart, and the digestive system, as well as being strongly anti-bacterial, anti-viral, and anti-fungal. They are also potent cancer-fighters.

Because atherosclerosis – the formation of fatty deposits in the arteries – is occurring earlier and earlier in the junk food generations, it is never too soon to start protecting children. Researchers have found that raw and also fried onions can pull down cholesterol levels in the blood.

QUICK FOOD IDEAS

If you've got the oven on, slice off the pointed tips across a whole bulb of garlic and put in the oven in a small ovenproof dish with a drizzle of oil for at least an hour. Then squeeze out wonderful garlic purée onto vegetables.

If you are baking potatoes, roast a whole unpeeled onion along with them and enjoy both with butter.

Wash and trim leeks, place them in an ovenproof dish with a drizzle of olive oil and lots of black pepper, and bake in a moderate oven until tender.

The onion family is more valued for it's protective phytochemicals than for high levels of nutrients. But scallions supply some vitamin C, and leeks **contain** vitamin C, folic acid, and potassium.

sweet bell peppers

Bell peppers come in rainbow colors, but children usually prefer the red, yellow, and orange ripe ones to the harder, less ripe green ones – and they are richer in antioxidants, too. Serve sticks of peppers with a dip (see page 149 for some ideas), in salads or in vegetable stir-fries.

A **rich source** of vitamin C and also of the protective antioxidant beta-carotene.

beets

Not, please, the horrible pickled things you buy in the supermarket. It's much better to choose the firm, raw, straight-from-the-ground variety, which, as its dramatic color suggests, is loaded with anthocyanins which are antioxidants and great cancer-fighters.

In Romany medicine, beets juice was used as a blood-builder for patients who were pale and run-down. And in Russia and Eastern Europe, it is used both to build up resistance and to treat convalescents after a serious illness. The fresh raw beets juice is a powerful blood-cleanser and tonic.

It has also been valued for centuries for its usefulness to the digestive system generally, and to the liver in particular – except when, as so often, it is soaked in hyperacid vinegars.

The popular French starter, crudités – a delicious combination of grated raw beets, raw carrots and perhaps paper-thin slices of cucumber, dressed with olive oil and lemon juice and garnished with chopped parsley – is a more powerful tonic for general health than a whole bottle of vitamin pills.

A **good source** of potassium and folic acid as well as of calcium.

green beans

When they are young and fresh in summer, green beans make a delicious vegetable contribution to a meal, whether you pick the big flat runner beans or the flat fava beans with the slippery skins. Green beans add color and interesting texture to meals, and they supply the beta-carotene and

vitamin C lacking in dried beans. Green beans can be eaten raw; especially fava beans which are best eaten when they are young and tender, when they make a delicious salad.

A **good source** of vitamin C, beta-carotene, potassium, and folic acid.

pumpkin

Winter squashes come in a huge variety of shapes and sizes, many of them, such as butternut and those interesting turban-shaped ones, being more widely available than in the past. But it is the Halloween pumpkin, a member of the winter squash family of vegetables that deserve to be eaten and enjoyed as food as well as being hollowed out as decorations for a party.

As their wonderful orange colors tell us, pumpkins are spectacularly rich in beta-carotene. It is not surprising, then, that in numbers of studies, the trio of pumpkin, carrots, and sweet potatoes give us the highest protection against lung cancer: regular consumption halved the risk

of contracting the disease, even for heavy smokers. If you smoke yourself, or if you cannot persuade teenagers who smoke not to, make sure you add plenty of these great vegetables to the menu as often as possible in your home.

In European folk medicine pumpkin is considered to be an especially good food for treating respiratory illnesses, as well as a soothing, protective food for the entire digestive tract. Add chunks of pumpkin to stews or make it into a cheerful winter soup (see Pumpkin Soup, page 133).

A **rich source** of beta-carotene.

super salads

Salads, with their fresh raw ingredients, put vitality into the daily menu. The tender young leaves, bright red tomatoes, cool cucumbers, and fresh herbs of summer bring sunshine straight to our tables, while crisp raw salads of celery and chicory, shredded cabbage, and grated carrot make wonderfully light salads for winter.

lettuces

Lettuces are more than just water. They contain good amounts of several nutrients, a little iodine, and even a modest amount of iron. As a rule, the darker the lettuce leaf, the higher its beta-carotene content. Iceberg lettuce is the least valuable nutritionally, but it does keep well and kids know it from fast-food restaurants, so don't ignore it. Even if you've only got a window box, growing lettuce is a good way to introduce children to growing and eating greens – try producing cut-and-come-again varieties like grand rapids, oak leaf, and cress.

A woman considering pregnancy should bear in mind that a 3½ oz/100g serving of lettuce provides more than a quarter of her daily folic acid requirement. And a lettuce sandwich at bedtime is a far healthier aid for insomnia than sleeping pills. The combined sedative effects of the lettuce and the tryptophan released by the digestion of carbohydrates contributes to a good night's sleep.

Sadly, all these nutritional values may be more than counter-balanced by chemical contamination: commercial lettuce crops may be sprayed dozens of times before they reach you. So, always be sure to wash lettuces well before eating them, or buy organic, if possible.

A **good source** of folic acid, potassium, and beta-carotene, and **contains** some vitamin C.

chicory

Wild chicory, the ancestor of both endive and celery, was highly regarded as a medicine derived from food in ancient Egypt, Greece, and Rome. Like most bitter foods, it is a liver stimulant and good digestive aid. Tear a few leaves into a green salad to give it crunch.

Chicory is more valuable for its phytochemicals than for its nutrients.

watercress

Hippocrates, who described watercress and its medicinal values in 460BC, built the world's first hospital next to a stream flowing with pure spring water so that he could grow fresh watercress for the benefit of his patients.

Watercress, like its relative the brightly colored nasturtium, contains a benzyl mustard oil – similar compounds give "bite" to the related horseradish and radish – which research has shown to be powerfully antibiotic. But, unlike conventional antibiotics, those in watercress are not only harmless to our intestinal flora, they are positively beneficial to the health of our intestines. So eat plenty of watercress and you will greatly enhance your natural resistance.

Dr Stephen Hecht, Professor of Cancer Prevention at the University of Minnesota, USA, has recently published a dramatic report on the importance of watercress in the prevention of lung cancer in smokers. Of course, he says, the best way to avoid lung cancer is to stop smoking, but for those who can't, chemoprevention in the form

QUICK FOOD IDEA

Combine chopped scallions, watercress, olive oil and lemon juice for a salad with "bite".

of 2oz/60g of watercress at three meals each day for three days will produce enough of the chemical phenethyl isothiocyanate, also known as gluconasturtin, to neutralize the important tobacco-specific lung carcinogen NNK. Phenethyl isothiocyanate is only released from watercress when it is chewed or chopped.

Because watercress is grown in water, it is specially important to wash it carefully before eating it to remove any waterborne parasites that may be present.

A **good source** of vitamins A, C, and E, the powerful antioxidants that protect against cardiovascular disease as well as cancers, and of iodine, essential for the proper functioning of the thyroid gland.

celery & celeriac

Both wild and cultivated varieties of celery have long been popular with herbalists, who use the leaves, stalks and seeds. Most children love the crunchy texture and mild flavor of celery and will happily nibble sticks of it, with or without a dip.

Celeriac is a turnip-rooted variety of celery but it is the bulbous round root which is eaten rather than the stalks. The two smell similar, but celeriac has a less pronounced flavor. Children enjoy eating celeriac grated into fine matchsticks, par-boiled, and served as salad with the addition of a creamy dressing.

Nutritionally and chemically, celery and celeriac are similar, but the white bulb of celeriac and

blanched white celery stalks do not contain beta-carotene, whereas dark green celery stalks do. Celeriac is a rich source of folate which makes it an excellent addition to salads for women planning pregnancy, and both vegetables supply vitamin C, potassium, and fiber.

Celery helps calm the nerves, wrote Hippocrates, and how right he was. Research in both China and Germany has demonstrated that essential oils extracted from celery seed have a powerful calming effect on the central nervous system.

Good sources of potassium; also **contain** reasonable levels of fiber and vitamin C, and some beta-carotene, if the green stalks are eaten.

tomatoes

Tomatoes are a fruit rather than a vegetable, and most children will enjoy their sweet freshness in the summer – as long as you buy only the brightest, ripest red tomatoes and forget about the insipid watery, flavorless things on sale for the rest of the year. Put a dish of tiny scarlet plum and cherry tomatoes on the table at the start of a meal: children will eat them happily. Tomatoes are extremely rich in antioxidants, especially carotenoids like beta-carotene and lycopene, as well as vitamins C and E, making them good protectors of the cardiovascular system and effective against some forms of cancer.

Tomato ketchup is super-rich in lycopene because the whole tomato, including its skin, goes into the ketchup. Organic tomato ketchup is now available – great for children's hamburgers.

QUICK FOOD IDEA

For a quick summer pasta, quarter ripe cherry tomatoes and stir them into cooked pasta with plenty of olive oil, some seasoning, and a handful of torn basil leaves.

Canned tomatoes lose very little of their nutrients, but they usually have added salt. If buying tomato juice or the traditional canned Italian tomatoes, choose low-salt varieties.

Sun-dried tomatoes are full of stored sunshine energy: add minced ones to enrich a tomato sauce for pasta, tomato soup or stews.

A **good source** of carotenoids, potassium, and vitamins C and E.

avocados

Avocados, like tomatoes, originated in South America. They are rich in healthy monounsaturated fats, making them especially valuable for children. Since avocados also contain compounds which stimulate the production of collagen, teenagers agonizing over pimples should eat them.

Weight-watching mothers who think avocados are fattening are misguided: half an avocado has the same number of calories as two apples and far more nutrients, so don't deprive your children or yourself on that basis.

Because the fats in avocados are very digestible and because they also contain anti-fungal and anti-bacterial chemicals, puréed avocado is an excellent food for invalids, people convalescing from illness, and sick children.

If you need to ripen avocados quickly, store them in a brown paper bag.

Chunks of avocado add a rich, creamy note to salads, or serve them as Guacamole, which most children enjoy, or in the popular Italian Tricolore Salad – slices of bright red tomatoes, cool green avocados, and creamy white mozzarella cheese, garnished with fresh basil leaves. There is also a tasty avocado dip on page 149.

A **good source** of essential fatty acids, potassium, vitamins A, C, and E, and iron.

super fruit

Fruit and vegetables are the most important health-giving and protective foods. To obtain a maximum of the good things in fruit, all children should eat at least two or three helpings every single day. Encouraging your children to eat fruit is a health investment that will last for the rest of their lives.

apples

"An apple a day keeps the doctor away." Indeed it does. Phenolic acids and flavonoids in the skins of apples have richly antioxidant qualities, inhibiting the growth of bowel- and liver-cancer cells, while apple juice has significant anti-viral properties. Eating five or more apples a week is thought to improve lung function, so encouraging children to eat apples could help keep them free of coughs, bronchitis, and even pneumonia and asthma.

And that's not all. Apples are rich in a soluble fiber – pectin – which helps the body to eliminate cholesterol and toxic heavy metals like lead and mercury. The soluble fiber also makes apples a good weapon against constipation.

Then, there's the malic and tartaric acids they contain: these help with the digestion of rich fatty foods. Apples are also good for treating diarrhea. Naturopaths recommend grated apple, left to turn brown and then mixed with a little honey, for this purpose. A diet including bananas, rice, apples, and dry toast is popular with doctors for the relief of diarrhea.

The sugar in apples is mostly fructose, a simple sugar that is broken down slowly and thus helps to keep blood sugar levels on an even keel. Modern apples contain very little vitamin C, but some of the old varieties like Stayman Winesap are not only delicious but good sources of the vitamin.

A **good source** of fiber, malic, and tartaric acids.

melon

Melons have a great taste and real benefits for health. They don't offer a lot in the way of classic nutrients like vitamins or minerals, though the deep orange varieties like canteloupe are antioxidant-rich. Melons are a cooling delicious treat in hot weather. A large slice of crisp-cool watermelon beats any can of carbonated drink for cool refreshment. All forms of melons are mildly laxative without being an irritant, making them good to give children who are constipated.

Contains some potassium, a small amount of iron, vitamin C, and folic acid.

citrus fruit

Oranges – at least when recently picked or freshly squeezed – have a high vitamin C content which accounts for much of their beneficial influence on our health. Vitamin C is enormously important in combating infection and preserving general health, and it plays a major part in helping the body absorb iron from other foods.

Oranges also contain beta-carotene, bioflavonoids (contained in pith and segment walls) which strengthen the walls of the tiny blood capillaries, and many other nutrients. Blood oranges, as you might expect, are particularly rich in protective antioxidants.

During the winter months when oranges are in season and at their juicy best, their vibrantly fresh taste is most welcome. And this season arrives just when the protective nutrients oranges contain are most valuable.

Too many children only see oranges in juice form: the whole orange, peeled and divided into neat little segments, is much more fun, as well as richer in fiber. And many children enjoy eating the flesh from crescents of oranges with the peeling still on.

As well as vitamin C, oranges also supply a whole spectrum of nutrition, including even protein, calcium, and iron. Their high potassium content makes them particularly useful to counter-balance the excess sodium in the potato chips popular with children.

The fruits, flowers, and peeling of both bitter and sweet oranges have long been used in herbal medicine. The peel contains hesperidine and limonene which are used in the treatment of chronic bronchitis. Tea made from the dried flowers is a mild sedative.

To obtain the best value from orange juice, be choosy about what you buy. Making your own from organic oranges just before you want to drink it is your best guarantee of maximum vitamin C content. The next best thing is freshly squeezed orange juice from your supermarket refrigeration section. But watch out: many of the products in the same-shaped bottles as fresh juice are "drinks" or "crushes" which may be full of sugar and may also have been pasteurized, which destroys much of the vitamin C content.

A **good source** of vitamin C, potassium, bioflavonoids, calcium, and folic acid.

Lemons are a whole medicine chest in themselves. Lemon juice with hot water and honey is the first thing you give to a child with a cold, a fever, or flu. Used in food preparation, lemons not only supply vitamin C but are also a wonderful anti-bacterial. They are friends to the digestive system: a thick slice of lemon in a glass of hot water is an instant remedy for a tummy upset. Used as a gargle or mouthwash, lemons are perfect for sore throats or mouth ulcers.

A **rich source** of vitamin C: add the juice of a lemon to salad dressings.

Grapefruit are also high in vitamin C – the deeper the color, the more vitamin C the fruit contains. One whole ruby grapefruit can contain a whole day's supply. The pith and skin between segments contain bioflavonoids so don't scrape them all away. The pink ones are sweeter, too, so are more palatable for children.

A **rich source** of bioflavonoids and vitamin C.

Clementines, mandarins, satsumas, and other varieties of small citrus fruit are all much less acidic than the bigger ones, are easier to peel and have few or no seeds, so children can manage them easily.

Rich sources of vitamin C and **good sources** of folate.

berries

Most children love berries, both for their dramatic colors and for their marvelous flavors. Modern research has revealed that colors and flavors are each produced by a host of nature's most powerful healing compounds. They protect against heart disease, cancer, urinary infections, painful joints, and skin disorders, and they are generally anti-viral, anti-bacterial, and anti-inflammatory.

For people who are susceptible to allergies, however, berries can cause allergic reactions (see pages 202–5). Also, berries, especially strawberries, contain salicylates, similar to salicylic acid which comprises aspirin, so people with aspirin intolerance should avoid them.

Strawberries

are rich in the soluble fiber pectin which helps in the body's elimination of cholesterol and toxic metals, such as lead, mercury, and cadmium. This, combined with their powerful antioxidant properties, makes them highly effective against heart and circulatory disease. There is also a growing body of evidence that these delicious berries have anti-viral properties, too.

Strawberries contain modest amounts of iron and the highest vitamin C level than any other of the widely available berries, 3½oz/100g of strawberries provide almost twice the body's vitamin C needs for a day. This extremely high vitamin C content contributes to the absorption of available iron, making strawberries useful in both the prevention and treatment of anemia and fatigue.

Having strawberries as a "medicine" doesn't need a spoonful of sugar to help it go down! These wonderful berries should be eaten on their own or at the start of a meal in order to achieve their therapeutic best. A few each day during the season is the cheapest, and most delicious, health insurance you can buy.

A **good source** of vitamin C; **contain** some iron.

Blackberries

are extremely rich in vitamin E (with wild berries having a higher concentration than the cultivated varieties) which is vital for the protection of the heart and arteries.

Their dramatic black color indicates the presence of valuable plant pigments called anthocyanins, which will help keep your children healthy. Add them – at the last minute to preserve their nutrients – to stewed apples, make them into delicious tarts or pies, or combine them with slices of crisp apple in a salad or a crumble. Too many children grow up without the faintest idea of where food comes from. Make sure yours enjoy the traditional fun of going out to the country on a summer afternoon to pick wild blackberries.

A **good source** of antioxidants, vitamins C and E, fiber, and potassium.

Raspberries,

like grapes, should be on every hospital menu. This delicious fruit is a rich source of vitamin C: 3½oz/100g provides 75 percent of the RDA. They are also a useful source of the soluble fiber, pectin, and contain small amounts of calcium, potassium, iron, and magnesium, all vital to the convalescent, as well as to those suffering from heart problems, fatigue, or depression – and all well-absorbed, thanks to their vitamin C content. This makes them the perfect food for a sickly child – or for children suffering from low spirits or tiredness.

Herbalists value raspberries for their cooling effect – useful in feverish conditions. Naturally astringent, raspberries can benefit the whole length of the digestive system, helping counter spongy, diseased gums, upset stomachs, and diarrhea along the way.

A **good source** of vitamin C, and useful source of iron, calcium, potassium, and magnesium.

Blueberries contain the anti-bacterial compounds anthocyanins, which have a tonic effect on blood vessels. They are are protective of the eyes, making them a true superfood for children who spend a lot of time in front of computer screens.

Blueberries are prized in traditional medicine as a treatment for cystitis and for diarrhea. In Scandinavian countries dried blueberry soup is a favorite treatment for diarrhea, as is chewing the dried berries.

Contain small amounts of vitamin C, vitamin B_1 and potassium: it is the natural chemicals they supply that make them medically valuable.

Cranberries are one of the few fruits native to North America. For centuries Native Americans used these extraordinary berries as both food and medicine. Thanks to the vitamin C in cranberries, early settlers from Europe avoided the terrors of scurvy, as did American whalers in later centuries. Today, no Thanksgiving dinner is complete without cranberry sauce served along with the turkey.

Science has recently validated the folk-remedy use of cranberry juice for both the prevention and treatment of cystitis, discovering a substance in cranberries that prevents infectious bacteria clinging to cells in the urinary tract and bladder. Cystitis can affect children as well as adults, and it is not uncommon in young girls, so it is worth including cranberries and juice regularly in your menus for preventative reasons.

Cranberries **contain** vitamin C, B vitamins, iron and other minerals.

Red currants are difficult to find fresh, but if you have a source for them, eat them in that form to obtain almost as much vitamin C as there is in oranges – 3½oz/100g will supply the recommended daily amount. This makes them valuable for improving the natural function of the immune system.

Although they lose some vitamin C when they are cooked, used as jams, jellies, juices, or stewed with other fruit, red currants can make an important contribution to the diet of a recovering invalid. The iron, fiber, and potassium in them are not lost during cooking.

Herbalists have traditionally recommended red currant juice as a refreshing and temperature-lowering drink for anyone with a fever.

A **good source** of vitamin C, potassium and antioxidants; **contain** iron and fiber.

cherries

Cherries are one of the few fruits not available for twelve months of the year so make the most of them while they are cheap and in season.

Because cherries have a reasonable potassium content and virtually no sodium, the fruit and the dried fruit stems are an extremely effective diuretic. They are excellent for children with a tendency to constipation, too. For these reasons, cherries are often regarded as a specially cleansing food. Their bright flushed yellow or deep red colors signal their protective anioxidant content.

Cherries are great for the lunchboxes of children old enough to manage the pits: put them in a small lidded carton so they don't get mashed over everything else in the box and there is somewhere convenient to put the pits.

A **good source** of bioflavonoids with some vitamin C, and potassium.

apricots

Wonderful ripe apricots, the true color of sunshine, should be enjoyed as often as possible, while they are cheap and in season. Whereas with most fruits fresh is best, apricots can be eaten fresh, cooked, or dried and their nutritional value remains enormous. Their massive content of carotenoids makes them highly protective of skin and eyesight and invaluable for general resistance. They are also one of nature's great anti-cancer foods. Dried apricots are an excellent source of fiber, iron, and

QUICK FOOD IDEA

Whizz soaked dried apricots in a blender with natural yogurt and honey.

healthy energy, so they deserve a place in every child's lunchbox.

A **good source** of beta-carotene and potassium; also **contain** iron and a little vitamin C.

bananas

Bananas are the perfect fast food, even coming in their own packaging. The starch in bananas is not easily digested, which is why children should only eat them ripe, when most of the starch has turned to sugar. This happens when the skin turns a speckled brown. Because ripe bananas are so easily digestible and the fiber in them is mainly of the soluble type, they are good for the treatment of both constipation and diarrhea, as well as helping to eliminate cholesterol from the body.

The high potassium content of bananas helps prevent cramps and combined with the easily available energy from the ripe fruit, makes them the ideal snack for active children. One banana contains a substantial amount of vitamin B_6, something that is often missing from children's diets and known to help in the prevention of depression, skin problems, and asthma.

A **good source** of potassium, as well as of vitamin B_6 and folic acid.

peaches & nectarines

Velvet-skinned peaches and smooth-skinned nectarines are sisters under their skins, and in fact they are both especially good for your skin – it is no coincidence that an admired complexion is described as "peaches-and-cream."

Nutritionally, there is little difference between peaches and nectarines. They both contain good amounts of vitamin C (nectarines slightly more, so that one will give you a day's requirements) small amounts of fiber, modest numbers of calories, some beta-carotene, and minerals. Dried peaches contain far more calories than fresh, but 3½oz/100g will

provide almost a day's requirement of iron and a third of your daily need for potassium. Forget canned peaches, especially those in high-calorie, high-sugar syrup, because nearly all the vitamin C is lost in the canning process.

Peaches and nectarines should be thoroughly washed before they are eaten, skin and all: don't encourage children to peel them since, as with many fruits, much of their nutritional value is concentrated in the skin.

A **good source** of vitamins A and C, and also **contain** iron.

pineapples

In Hawaii, chunks of juicy pineapple are eaten by old and young as a delicious cure for digestive problems. Scientists explain that this is because the fresh fruit is rich in an enzyme, bromelain, which can digest many times its own weight of protein in a few minutes and only breaks down food and dead tissue, leaving our intestines undamaged. The juice of fresh pineapples, used as an instant gargle, is also an effective folk medicine for sore throats and was once a favorite herbal remedy for diphtheria. This is because pineapples contain compounds with marked antibiotic and anti-inflammatory effects.

Some of these compounds, though not the enzyme bromelain, probably survive the processing that produces commercial juice or canned fruit. But for maximum healing potential, fresh ripe pineapple or freshly extracted juice must be your first choice. Eating fresh pineapple or drinking pineapple juice is a good remedy for bruising sports injuries, such as falls, kicks, or knocks. This is because the enzyme bromelain breaks down the accumulating blood in the injured area that causes the bruising to appear.

When choosing a pineapple, choose one that feels heavy for its size as this is a good guide to quality. Forget the old superstition that a pineapple is only ripe if you can tug a leaf out easily – it's not a true test.

A **good source** of fiber, and **contain** vitamin C.

QUICK FOOD IDEAS

Pineapple Iced Pops: whizz fresh pineapple in a blender or food processor and freeze in popcicle molds. Better than ice cream for a sore throat.

Pineapple Sorbet: combine puréed pineapple with sugar syrup. Freeze, stir, and freeze again.

kiwis

Kiwis contain almost twice as much vitamin C as oranges and more fiber than an apple. One kiwi will give you twice as much vitamin C as the recommended minimum daily intake. This vitamin C content remains very stable; although there are some losses soon after harvesting, 90 percent of it is still present after six months in storage.

Kiwis are particularly rich in potassium, a mineral of which American diets, with their junk food high in sodium, can be dangerously short. The average kiwi supplies about 250mg of potassium, but only about 4mg of sodium.

When buying kiwis, avoid the rock-hard ones and choose those that are soft enough to yield to gentle pressure. They can be stored for several days in the refrigerator and should not be peeled until just before they are to be eaten.

The fiber content of kiwis and their particular type of mucilage make them an excellent, but extremely gentle, laxative, ideal for children who are often constipated from eating too much junk food.

A **good source** of vitamin C and potassium; also **contain** vitamin E.

QUICK FOOD IDEA

Once they've tried them, most kids will adore kiwis. Encourage them by putting one in an eggcup, slicing off the top, and letting children eat it with a spoon just like a boiled egg.

exotic fruits

As you would expect, fruits from sun-drenched tropical climes are high in protective antioxidants. As well as insisting on sunscreens and floppy hats, it makes sense to give children extra protection by giving them an abundance of these succulent fruits – where better to eat a mango than on the beach?

Mangoes are a delicious and health-giving treat, packed full of nutrients. One average-size fruit gives the minimum daily need of vitamin C, two- thirds of vitamin A, nearly half vitamin E, and almost a quarter of fiber, as well as useful contributions of potassium, iron, and nicotinic acid. It's this great combination of antioxidants in a very easily digested form that should put the mango on everybody's weekly shopping list.

In their native India, mangoes are part of the way of life and are eaten all year round. In the hot season drinks are made from pulped mangoes to replace body fluids. Panna is made from pulped mangoes strained with salt, molasses, and cumin, and mango chutney is served with spiced dishes.

Good source of vitamins A, C, and E; also **contain** potassium, iron, and some B vitamins.

QUICK FOOD IDEA

When mangoes are cheap and plentiful, use them for juice, milkshakes, sauces and iced pops.

HEALTH WARNING

Mango peel can be highly irritant. Anyone who has previously been sensitized by mangoes can suffer a severe reaction. Even cutting the flesh with the knife you used to peel the mango can cause sufficient contamination to represent a hazard. If dealing with large numbers of mangoes, be sure to wear kitchen gloves.

Papayas are nutritionally very important. They are a rich source of beta carotene, which makes them excellent for treating skin problems. An average-size papaya supplies twice the minimum daily need of vitamin C, so the fruit helps boost the body's immune defence mechanisms. It also supplies well over a quarter of vitamin A. Because a fully ripe papaya needs no cooking, it can be quickly puréed or mashed to make an excellent and convenient first food for babies.

The most important constituent of the papaya is the enzyme papain, which is a great aid to digestion. In South American cooking, meat is often wrapped in papaya leaves to tenderize it.

A **good source** of vitamins C and A, beta-carotene, and fiber.

Guavas are an extremely rich source of vitamin C: one average-size fruit supplies five days' worth of the minimum requirement. There are many varieties, in a great range of sizes and flesh colors. The pink-fleshed varieties are richer in vitamin C than those with white flesh and the content is at its peak in green mature fruits.

Canned guavas can lose up to a third of their vitamin C content during processing, but are still an excellent source of the vitamin and retain the fiber content.

Guava has become popular as a drink but it is sold heavily sweetened as guava nectar.

A **rich source** of vitamin C; a **good source** of beta-carotene, phosphorus, calcium, and the B vitamin nicotinic acid.

QUICK FOOD IDEA

Fresh guava purée added to a carton of natural yogurt makes an exceptionally health-giving and delicious "shake." Rich in calcium, intestinal-friendly bacteria, vitamins and fiber, it is a really nutritious addition to breakfast.

grapes

Every child's favorite fruit – especially the seedless varieties – but make sure they are well washed. Grapes are uniquely nourishing, strengthening, cleansing and regenerative. They are useful for anemia and for fatigue.

Grapes contain enormous numbers of protective compounds called polyphenols; most of these are concentrated in the skin, and there are more of them in purple than in white grapes, which is why red wine has earned its reputation as protection for the heart when drunk in moderation. The same compounds help prevent cancer, too.

A **good source** of potassium; also **contain** vitamin C.

dried fruit

Dates are mostly sold semi-dried, although
fresh dates are also now available. Avoid the ones in gift boxes, which are heavily coated with sugar.

Fresh dates provide 96 calories per 3½oz/100g, but 3½oz/100g dried dates will give you around 250 calories. Fresh dates contain modest amounts of vitamin C, but there is virtually none in the dried variety.

It is the minerals in dates which are most interesting, especially their iron content. The amount of iron is totally dependent on the variety of date. One or two date varieties are very poor sources of iron, but the vast majority make highly significant contributions.

Their high iron content together with their easily available energy make dates an excellent nutrient for those suffering from anaemia and illnesses which produce chronic fatigue. They are a healthier sweet snack than chocolates or cookies.

A **rich source** of iron and potassium; **contain** fiber and some B vitamins, including folic acid.

Prunes, which are dried plums, have an
unfortunate reputation among children: perhaps if kids weren't told so often that prunes are good for them, they might like them better. As part of a mixed compote of fruit they are good to eat and a great source of instant energy, iron, fiber, and a range of vitamins including A and B_6.

Prunes' well-known laxative action is due to a natural chemical that gently stimulates the bowel muscle. Since constipation is common in children, and irritant purgatives should be avoided, a few prunes occasionally will help avoid problems.

A **good source** of fiber, potassium, iron, and vitamins A, niacin, and B_6.

Golden raisins, black raisins, and currants have all the nutritional benefits of
grapes concentrated in them, making them a wonderful store of instant energy for children and adults alike.

These dried fruits are spectacularly rich in potassium, a mineral useful for counteracting the high salt content of many fast foods and commercial breakfast cereals.

The perfect snack is a package of raisins, particularly when mixed with fresh unsalted nuts (over five-year-olds only) to provide protein as well as energy.

A **rich source** of potassium; a **good source** of iron, fiber, and some B vitamins.

HEALTH WARNING

Non-organic dried fruits are treated with the preservative sulfur dioxide. Some are coated in mineral oil, too. Wash them carefully in warm water to remove both ingredients.

super legumes

One of the **first food crops** ever cultivated, beans originated in the Middle East thousands of years ago. **Dried beans** and other **legumes** are basic foods and essential in the diets of people all over the world today, being rich in **body-building** protein as well as in sustaining complex carbohydrates.

dried beans

A huge variety of dried beans is available today. There are the white beans of Western traditional cooking; the dark red kidney beans that are essential to Chili con carne; the small black beans of Tex-Mex cooking; and the tiny green mung beans – most digestible of all the beans – of Indian cooking. Black-eyed beans, aduki, pinto and navy beans, and those speckled Italian borlotti beans are other members of this huge food family.

Ounce for ounce, beans contain almost as much protein as a good steak, with much less fat – beans are very low in fat – and lots of the soluble fiber that takes care of the heart and circulation. And they're high in complex carbohydrates which supply the best kind of energy for active children.

So, if you're in such a rush that all you have time to do for the kids' supper is heat up a can of baked beans in tomato sauce (sugar-free are best) and toast some bread to put them on, don't feel guilty: you're giving them a really nourishing meal.

Canning has turned beans into wonderful fast food. But canned beans can never have quite the authentic flavor and fresh taste of beans you have soaked and cooked yourself, and, although you need to plan bean-feasts well ahead, you'll only need to spend minutes on actual preparation.

You can also speed up the process. Instead of soaking the beans overnight, put them in a pan with enough water to cover them by 5in/13cm. Bring to a boil and boil rapidly for 2 minutes, then cover the pan, remove from the heat, and let them soak for least an hour – more if you have the time. Drain the beans and start cooking them.

Soaking beans overnight is useful because the process helps break down the compounds that give beans their notorious reputation for causing gas. Many herbs and spices, including winter savory and parsley, also counter the flatulence beans can produce.

Rich sources of B-complex vitamins; the minerals calcium, iron, magnesium, and zinc; and protein and soluble fiber.

QUICK FOOD IDEAS

Baked beans on toast

Tuna and beans: flake canned tuna into well-rinsed canned white beans; dress with plenty of olive oil, lemon juice, pepper, and a little salt; garnish with onion rings and chopped parsley.

chickpeas

Like beans, chickpeas need long soaking before being cooked in plenty of water: 4 cups/1.5 liters for 8oz/250g dried chickpeas. Chickpeas add a special nutty flavor to spicy stews; they make delicious salads, and chickpea flour is used in India to make savory pancakes or to wrap around meat or vegetables like tortillas. Chickpeas are also a key ingredient of hummus.

A **rich source** of iron, calcium, magnesium, fiber and protein.

lentils

Lentils may have been the first-ever cultivated crop and there are many varieties of them, usually named after their color, which can be green, red-orange, yellow, brown, or black. To get the best value from their iron content, lentils need to be eaten with salads or vegetables rich in vitamin C so that the iron can be absorbed. They need no presoaking and only about 35–40 minutes cooking. They can give body to warming soups and stews. Serve them with roasts and add them to salads.

A **good source** of B vitamins, fiber and protein; high in iron, calcium, zinc, and other minerals.

split peas

Dried peas have been used for thousands of years, made into the solid sustaining soups of medieval peasants, the pea pudding of English cooking, the aromatic yellow purées of Greece, or dressed with oil and lemon and served as a meze with pita bread. They are sold skinned and split, so they don't need soaking: cook them for 45–50 minutes.

A **good source** of protein and fiber.

soy beans

Soy beans are the source of such familiar foods as soy drink (also called soy milk), tofu, tempeh, soy sauce, miso, soy oil, and TVP (textured vegetable protein). Like all beans, they are great sources of fiber, protein and some minerals. Soy beans also contain plant chemicals called isoflavones which mimic the action of natural estrogens. However, studies have shown that those who eat soy regularly do not have a lower incidence of hormone-related cancers, such as breast or prostate cancers, and heart disease, than the West. However, isoflavones are found in all legumes, and too much soy can cause thyroid problems unless, like the Japanese, you eat plenty of seaweed; studies of people who eat diets rich in any of the legumes also show up lower rates of cancer and heart disease. Other studies, too, suggest that it is lifelong regular consumption of these legumes that promotes protection.

Tempeh and tofu are good meat-substitutes in stir-fries or soups; organic tamari soy sauces add a great jolt of flavor to soups, rice dishes, and stews, and miso may help protect against radiation.

A **good source** of protein and fiber.

super nuts & seeds

Think of nuts and you think of a cheap and handy snack, a little package of something to nibble. But to our hunter-gatherer ancestors, nuts were far more than a mere snack: with their high fat and protein content, they were a diet staple, and particularly useful since they were easy to store and transport – when they weren't being eaten straight from the tree.

Nuts are an excellent source of protein, which makes them a must for vegetarian children. Many nuts contain more protein than beef, and, whereas beef comes laced with saturated fat, the fats in fresh nuts are mono- or polyunsaturated, which favor healthy hearts. Nuts are good sources of antioxidants and they're high in fiber – essential for general health.

So, it is hardly surprising that a famous Seventh-Day Adventist study, which has been in progress since the mid-twentieth century, shows that people who eat nuts more than four times a week have only half the number of heart attacks of those who eat them only once a week.

Allergic reactions to peanuts and to other nuts, which can in some cases be fatal, are becoming alarmingly common among children (see pages 202 and 204). The widespread use of peanut oil in processed foods and baked goods, and even in nursing mothers' nipple cream, is believed to be responsible for this.

Make sure that nuts are fresh – straight from the shell, if possible – because their high fat content means they easily turn rancid when shelled. Buy nuts in small quantities in their shells or whole rather than broken, and eat them up quickly. Store them in the freezer: they defrost quickly.

For maximum absorption of their mineral content, eat nuts with vitamin C-rich fruits and salads, or toast them lightly. As for those tempting little packages of nuts, avoid them except as treats: they are usually very high in salt and in fat, too.

Nuts are **rich sources** of protein and fiber and of the minerals calcium, magnesium, potassium, iron, and zinc; and they are **good sources** of B-complex vitamins, except vitamin B_{12};

Seeds – future foods – are little powerhouses of nutrition. Tossed in a little hot oil for just seconds, they make delicious crunchy additions to salads; roasting or dry-frying seeds helps release their aromatic essential oils, thus increasing their flavor. Better still, teach your children how to sprout them – and grains and legumes too – because then their nutritional value rises dramatically.

Seeds are **rich sources** of protein, essential fatty acids, and several minerals.

HEALTH WARNING

Because of the increasing incidence of allergic reaction to nuts – especially peanuts – among children, allergy specialists suggest that children whose families have a history of allergies should not be given nuts to eat in any form until they are five or six years old. Children under three years old should not be given whole nuts because they could easily choke on them.

almonds

Almonds are such a richly nutritious, body-building food that five or six are as many as anyone should eat at a meal. Almonds are 20 per cent protein by weight, and weight for weight they have a third more protein than eggs. A great energy food, they also contain an oil that is particularly bland and soothing: almond milk used to be given to babies as one of their first foods. For children who have a problem with dairy foods, almond milk, which can be bought in some health-food stores, is an excellent substitute for cow's milk with breakfast cereal. To skin almonds, dunk them in boiling water for half a minute, then drain and rub the skins off between thumb and finger – a job even young children can do to help. Bought ground almonds are sometimes adulterated with other nuts, or have a trace of bitter almond – better to make your own in a food processor.

A **good source** of protein, B vitamins, and zinc, iron, calcium, and magnesium.

walnuts

Much the best way to enjoy these is by cracking the fresh nuts to dig out that tasty little kernel, a healthy way to end a meal. They are also great in salads, such as the classic Waldorf Salad.

A **good source** of protein, omega-3 fatty acids, potassium, zinc, some B vitamins and vitamin E.

chestnuts

The least fatty and the starchiest of the nuts – flour can be made from them – but richly nutritious as well. All children love the fuss and messy fingers of that wonderful mid-winter treat, roast chestnuts.

Contain vitamin E, potassium, vitamin B_6, and omega-3 fatty acids.

brazil nuts

Eat just one Brazil nut and you've probably taken in one day's supply of your body's requirement for the mineral selenium, a key player in the immune system, and a vital antioxidant which helps protect our hearts. Soils dedicated to intensive farming are likely to be depleted of their selenium content, but there's plenty of this key mineral in the soils of the Amazon rain forest where these nuts are grown. Brazil nuts are high in fat so they turn rancid very quickly: buy only small amounts at a time.

A **good source** of selenium and protein.

peanuts

The world's most popular snack is not actually a nut, but a legume. Peanuts can be eaten raw straight from those funny shells, or roasted, and most children love peanut butter. They are rich in protein, quite low in fat, and filled with other nutrients, so peanut butter is a very healthy food for children, but look for brands without extra salt or added sugar. (For peanuts allergy, see page 204.)

A **good source** of protein, vitamin D, fibre, magnesium, iron, and zinc.

pistachio nuts

These should be eaten from the shell when they are fresh – if only for the fun of cracking open their tough little shells to get at the green kernels inside. Pistachios have the lowest fat content of any nut, and much of the fat they do have is healthy monounsaturated fat. Their delicious flavor does not need enhancing by roasting or salting: try to eat the unsalted kind.

A **good source** of healthy fats, plus protein and significant amounts of four vital minerals: magnesium, calcium, iron and potassium.

pine nuts

The softest and most delicate of all the nuts, pine nuts are an essential ingredient in the Italian pasta sauce and pesto. They can also be tossed in a little oil for salads, or added to savory rice dishes.

A **good source** of protein, magnesium, iron, zinc, potassium, and vitamin E.

cashew nuts

This delicious nut is always sold shelled and roasted to destroy the film of caustic oil between the two layers of its shell. Avoid the salted ones and choose plain roasted. Cashews are high in healthy heart-protecting monounsaturated fats.

A **good source** of protein, potassium and B vitamins, including folate.

hazelnuts

Deliciously crunchy hazelnuts are rich in the B vitamin thiamin, deficiency of which can make people of any age feel low and lethargic. And they supply the omega-3 fatty acids needed for balance in our diets.

A **good source** of protein, fiber, thiamin, magnesium, and vitamin E.

pumpkin seeds

Buy them all ready shelled and dry-roast them in a non-stick pan to add to salads, or as a crunchy snack: they are an exceptionally good source of zinc and vital for our immune systems, our skin, and efficient brain functioning.

A **good source** of zinc, protein, fiber, iron, magnesium, and potassium,

sesame seeds

Children love the nutty taste of these tiny, light-brown seeds: add them to muesli, toast them and sprinkle on salads, add to rice dishes, or mix into yogurt with honey for a super-snack. Do not buy sesame seeds that are an even pale-cream color – they have been chemically hulled. The calcium in sesame seeds is easily assimilated.

A **good source** of protein, calcium, zinc, iron, and potassium.

sunflower seeds

These go rancid very quickly, when they turn yellow, brown, or black instead of their pearly gray: avoid sunflower seeds so colored. Eat them up soon after you buy them. A high-protein snack, they are a useful source of vitamin E and important B vitamins.

A **good source** of protein, iron, calcium, and vitamin E.

QUICK FOOD IDEAS

Toasted or tossed in a teaspoon of olive oil, nuts can give a satisfying crunch to salads.

Make your own mixed-nut butter as a change from peanuts: combine two or three different nuts – perhaps cashews, pistachios, almonds, and/or hazelnuts – and drop them into a blender with a little olive oil.

Ground almonds make a great topping for crumbles, either on their own or added to the usual flour-based crumbles. Buy ground almonds in small amounts and use them up within a few days, or make your own in a food processor from whole almonds.

super grains

Unrefined grains have been the staple diet of some of the hardiest and healthiest races on the planet. Richly nourishing, whole grains are an essential part of any child's diet, supplying **protein** for body-building, **carbohydrate** for energy, **fiber** for a healthy heart and digestive system, and essential **fats**, **vitamins**, and **minerals**.

wheat

Today, much of the world's bread is made from wheat, including the chapattis of India and the pita of the Middle East. The husk or bran of wheat is rich in fiber, minerals such as iron and calcium, B vitamins and important trace elements including chromium, which helps stabilize blood sugar levels (see page 14). The germ of the wheat is a nutritional treasury, supplying antioxidant vitamin E, B vitamins, minerals, and healthy fats. The white flour widely used for bread, cakes, cookies, and other processed foods loses much of its goodness, including zinc, magnesium, vitamin B_6, and vitamin E, when the germ and fiber-rich outer husk, or bran, are stripped out in milling. Thus, only whole wheat flour, which is milled from the whole grain, can claim to be a true superfood.

Bulgur or **cracked wheat,** a Middle Eastern favorite, retains much of the goodness of whole wheat. Since the grains are already roasted, bulgur can make a nourishing salad after a simple rinse and 10-minute soaking. Add extra-virgin olive oil, massive amounts of mint and parsley, and chopped tomatoes to make the Lebanese salad Tabbouleh; or serve it with Roasted Vegetables (see page 174) for a satisfying supper.

Sprouted wheat is tremendously rich nutritionally and fresh **wheatgerm,** the germ of the grain extracted during milling, is a superfood for growing children, packed with B vitamins and essential fatty acids. Store fresh wheatgerm in the refrigerator and use it up quickly, sprinkled on cereals or in place of breadcrumbs in cooking.

Semolina, made from the hard outer part of wheat, is used in the making of **couscous** and **pasta,** both great superfoods, providing children of all ages with lots of slow-release energy.

Note: see Allergies (page 204) for the problems some children have with eating wheat-based foods.

QUICK FOOD IDEAS

Whole wheat pancakes served with apple purée.

Whole wheat pita pizzas, brushed with oil, topped with sliced tomatoes, a pinch of dried oregano, seasoning, and grated cheese, then grilled.

Sprouted wheat with hummus and tomato slices in sandwiches.

rice

Rice is the foundation of the diet for half of humanity, and for centuries it was eaten with only the inedible outer husk removed. This unrefined rice is a low fat, very easily digested food supplying lots of energy and useful amounts of some B vitamins.

Brown rice, the whole natural grain with its bran, is more nutritious than white rice and helps stabilize blood sugar levels. Brown rice takes longer to cook than white, but is much harder to overcook. To prepare, wash it well and put in a saucepan with a teaspoon of vegetable bouillon powder and enough water to cover by about ½ inch deep. Cover the pan tightly and cook for about 40 minutes. It can also be cooked in a casserole in a low oven. Brown basmati rice, with a delicious nutty flavor, takes about 25 minutes to cook.

White rice, universally eaten today, is polished to remove the outer husk and the germ as well, thus stripping it not only of all its fiber and 60 percent of its mineral content, but most of its vitamins too, including almost all the B vitamin thiamin, which we need for the digestion of carbohydrates. "Par-boiled" or "converted" rice has some of these nutrients driven back into it by steaming.

Rice water, made by cooking 1oz/30g whole rice in 5 cups/1.2 liters water and then straining it, is a traditional remedy for diarrhea.

QUICK FOOD IDEAS

Cooked brown rice mixed with apple purée is an old country favorite for a soothing and sustaining supper.

If you have leftover cooked rice, fry mixed vegetables – carrots, onions, leeks, cabbage, zucchini, tomatoes, sliced and diced small – in a wok, then add the cooked rice and a cupful of hot vegetable stock. Cover and simmer for 20 minutes.

Use up cooked rice in croquettes: add grated cheese, chopped parsley, and a beaten egg to the rice; form into croquettes, dust with flour, and fry.

See also Brown Rice Four Ways (page 173).

millet

The only grain that is a complete protein, millet is a richly nutritious food for growing children, low in starch and very easily digested. It contains more iron than any other cereal, and plenty of magnesium. It is also high in silicon, a mineral needed for strong bones, teeth and nails, and healthy hair. Since it is gluten-free, millet can be eaten by children sensitive to the gluten in grains (see page 204). It should always be washed several times under cold water and drained before cooking. Try a millet pilaf as a change from rice as a savoury side dish: put 5 cups/1.2 liters water in a pan with a tablespoon of butter and a little salt, and bring to a boil. Add 8oz/250g millet (weighed before washing), bring back to a boil, lower the heat, cover tightly, and cook for 30–40 minutes, stirring occasionally. The mixture will be thick and have the consistency of cooked cereal.

To prepare millet like a breakfast muesli, put a tablespoon of millet in a bowl, add a cupful of milk and a spoonful of honey. Mix together thoroughly, cover, and refrigerate overnight. In the morning, add more milk if necessary, and chopped bananas, berries, or grated apple. Millet is an ingredient in the famous health food Five-Grain Kruska (see page 123).

oats

For centuries oats were eaten as a staple food throughout northern and eastern Europe, often in the form of a simple cooked cereal. Until the nineteenth century oats were the mainstay of the Scottish country diet, too, and according to one Scottish physician they produced "a big-boned, well-developed, and mentally energetic race."

Rolled oats and **oatmeal**, the milled grain, are both high in protein, rich in minerals including zinc, iron, calcium and magnesium, and they pack in enough B vitamins to rank as a first-class remedy for nerves and exhaustion – just the food for stressed-out teenagers. They're also a rare source of the omega-3 essential fatty acids.

The fiber in oats interests cardiologists, too: in studies at Kentucky University, high cholesterol levels nose-dived when a diet rich in oats was eaten. And before insulin was discovered, one of the few effective treatments for diabetes was the

"oat-cure": oats have a remarkably stabilizing effect on blood-sugar levels.

One way and another, in fact, this warming and nourishing food will send children off to school full of energy and keep them going all morning.

QUICK FOOD IDEAS

Cooked cereal, properly made with fresh oatmeal, eaten with honey and a spoonful of cream.

Fresh trout or mackerel rolled in rolled oats, then fried.

When making bread, substitute 1oz/30g oatmeal for 1oz/30g of every 1lb/500g flour.

2 oatcakes (see recipe page 158) with a hunk of cheese, a glass of milk, and an apple adds up to a perfectly balanced quick snack.

corn

Pre-Colombian America feasted on this grain from South America and used every part of it for medicine. But when corn became the staple diet of the very poor in the South and in parts of Europe, thousands fell sick with pellagra, the deficiency disease caused by lack of vitamin B_3. For this reason, corn should be served with good sources of vitamin B_3, such as eggs, tuna, or milk. This defect apart, corn is still a delicious user-friendly food that children eat with gusto, especially messy, delicious corn on the cob with plenty of butter. Sweetcorn, fresh or frozen, provides more protein than potatoes, plenty of fiber, useful vitamins, and minerals.

The flour from corn is made into polenta, a near-solid deep yellow creamy food that Italians love to combine with roast chicken or dark

aromatic game stews. Popcorn is a healthy snack, easily made at home. Both cornflour and popcorn are made from unmilled corn.

QUICK FOOD IDEAS

Corn with tuna, sliced tomatoes, parsley, and basil, and French dressing for a quick salad.

As a side-dish: melt 1 tablespoon of butter in a saucepan, add a package of frozen corn, stir, cover, and let heat through for 5–6 minutes. Season and add chopped parsley.

To make salt-free popcorn, heat a little oil in a large pan, drop in popping corn, cover tightly, and wait for the music!

barley

Probably the oldest of all cultivated grains, barley is rich in useful minerals, with particularly high levels of bone-building calcium and plenty of B vitamins. In ancient Rome it was valued as a particularly strengthening food, fed to gladiators in training. Tell that to your 10-year-old son! Grains of barley are unrefined: eat them in preference to pearl barley, which cooks much faster but has lost a lot of its goodness in refining. Barley is an ingredient in Five-Grain Kruska (see page 123). Herbalists value barley for its uniquely soothing action throughout the length of the digestive tract, and it makes a nourishing and soothing drink for children laid low with tummy upsets. Most children, well or sick, like Lemon Barley Water.

rye

Rye flour makes coarse and heavy black bread, and the rye bread you buy in bakeries is usually half rye and half wheat flour for this reason. But rye is a wonderfully warming grain for winter – survival food for millions of Russian peasants through long hard winters – and is rich in fiber. It is also particularly low in gluten. Rye crispbread is a must for the kitchen pantry.

buckwheat

Buckwheat is actually a seed, but it has always been used in grain-like ways – chiefly as kasha, the cooked cereal-like food eaten throughout eastern Europe right down to the steppes of Russia. According to the US Department of Agriculture, the protein in buckwheat is complete, and as valuable as that in meat. It is also a rich source of magnesium and zinc as well as in a flavonoid called rutin, which helps keep the walls of the tiniest blood capillaries strong and elastic. Buckwheat has a fairly strong flavor which some children may not like. To persuade them to try it, make the Buckwheat Crêpes on page 148.

ancient grains

Growing numbers of people are sensitive to certain common foods – over 35 million people in the US, according to the National Institute of Health – and wheat is one of the most frequently cited allergens. Diversifying your diet by eating from a wider range of grains makes obvious sense: the more so since some of the ancient grains are much richer in protein, minerals, and fiber than modern wheat. A growing range of these grains, as wholegrain flours, cereals, and mixes for baked goods, are becoming available. Look for the following grains in health-food stores.

Kamut has been raised in Montana from a package of grain shipped from Egypt in the 1970s. Clinical trials conducted in Chicago for the International Food Allergy Association indicated that 70 percent of those severely allergic to wheat could tolerate kamut. This ancient cousin of durum wheat is lighter and softer in baked goods than whole wheat flour. It is also higher in protein and richer in almost every mineral.

Quinoa, like buckwheat, is a seed rather than a grain. The Incas cultivated it and thought highly of it, perhaps because of its high protein content, as well as its slightly smoky taste. It is available in health-food stores as a wholegrain or flour. To make a creamy cooked cereal, add one part of well-washed grain to two parts water in a pan, bring to a boil, cover, lower the heat, and simmer for 12–15 minutes. Fluff with a fork and serve with butter and chopped fresh herbs as a savoury pilaf. Add quinoa to nourishing winter soups.

Spelt was the grain of the Roman armies, and highly regarded in the Middle Ages as particularly nourishing and ideal for building strong bodies and healthy blood. It is actually richer in protein than today's wheat, has more minerals, and special sugars that help boost resistance. Spelt wholegrain flour makes delicious bread and can be substituted for wheat flour in baking.

Another bonus is that many wheat-sensitive people find they have no problem with spelt.

Amaranth, which has a slightly nutty flavor, was cultivated by the Aztecs and the Incas. It deserves to be on any family shopping list, since this ancient grain is a whopping 16 percent protein – compared to wheat's 10 percent or the 7 percent of rice. It is also a rich source of calcium and has more than three times the iron content of wheat.

super meat

Before grains and legumes were extensively cultivated, meat, fish and fowl were our early ancestors' most reliable source of protein. In today's varied diet, meat still offers valuable protein and other important nutrients for growing children. Of all the areas where "organic" is really important, meat for children must come first, to avoid the risks of growth hormones, neurotoxic chemicals, and antibiotics.

beef

Beef has traditionally been one of the most highly sought-after of all meats. There is no denying the nutritional benefit of beef. It supplies most of our dietary needs apart from fiber, though some constituents are present only in small amounts.

The way beef is cooked is nutritionally important. Trimming visible fat before cooking reduces total fat in such dishes as stews and casseroles. Cuts should be roasted on a trivet so that the fat drips through into the pan and can be removed before making gravy from the residual juices. Steaks and chops should be cooked in the same way.

Beefburgers made at home from lean ground steak are great for kids, but commercially produced ones are inevitably high in fat. A standard burger isn't bad at only ⅓oz/9g of fat, but a quarter-pounder has about ¾oz/20g, rising to a massive 2oz/63g in a double 4oz/125g burger with cheese and all the trimmings. And that's without the fries!

Beef in small quantities is a good constituent of a normal mixed diet, but advice from the WHO and the Harvard School of Public Health suggests it should only be eaten a few times a month or, if more frequently, in very small amounts.

A **rich source** of protein, and a **good source** of calcium, vitamin C, and folate.

Note: not all children will eat organ meats, but beef and calf liver (and lamb and pork liver, too) are extremely rich sources of nutrients, especially easily absorbed iron and vitamins A and B_{12}, so offering liver to children is always worth trying.

HEALTH WARNING

Undercooked beefburgers may contain harmful bacteria. One strain, E.coli 0157:H7 VTEC, gets in at the time of slaughtering and, when the beef is ground, is distributed throughout the finished product. This particular strain can cause serious illness and even death. Thorough cooking until there is no trace of pink in the meat or juices is essential to destroy this E.coli bacterium.

lamb

Spring lamb is always more tender and has a lower fat content than older sheep, though modern breeds are all lower in fat generally. The amount of fat that you get with your lamb depends on the cut, how it is cooked, and the part you eat: neck fillet and leg are lower-fat cuts. Ideally, the fat should be removed before cooking and any that's left on the meat will protect it in cooking but should not be eaten.

A **rich source** of protein, easily absorbed iron, and zinc, and B vitamins.

pork (& bacon)

There is a popular misconception that pork is a "fatty" meat, whereas in fact modern breeds produce pork which contains less fat than beef or lamb and very little more than chicken – if you don't eat the skin.

There's no doubt, though, that pork is an extremely good source of several nutrients, while the iron it contains is heme iron, which is much more easily absorbed and used by the body than that of other meats. Some of the chemicals used in producing ham and bacon are known to be carcinogenic if consumed in excess, particularly the nitrites. Both products are also high in salt and should be eaten sparingly.

A **rich source** of thiamin (vitamin B_1), niacin, riboflavin (vitamin B_2), and zinc; and a **good source** of vitamin B_6, phosphorus, and iron.

rabbit

Delicious, delicately flavoured, high in protein and low in fat, cuts of rabbit can be broiled or sautéed, but rabbit stew is the traditional and best method of cooking. Children sometimes have problems with the bones so these should be removed. To compensate for the rabbit's lack of many nutrients, use plenty of root vegetables in the stew and serve it with a large salad.

A **rich source** of protein; very low in fat; also **contains** minerals and B vitamins.

venison

Venison, farmed rather than wild, is making a comeback in supermarkets, so if your children are adventurous with their eating, why not give venison a try? Flavour and texture are superb and it contains only a third of the calories and half the fat of beef, and even less than chicken.

Prime cuts should be cooked very hot and for just enough time to be medium rare. Otherwise, marinate before cooking. Red wine, oil and herbs are common marinades and buttermilk is a favorite. A slow-cooked venison hotpot with lots of vegetables and a hunter's campfire recipe in which it is cooked in coffee and cider vinegar are both wonderful.

A **rich source** of protein and ultra-low in fat; also **contains** zinc, iron, and B vitamins.

super poultry

All poultry is a terrific source of protein, B vitamins and minerals, making it an ideal food for growing children, a real boost during periods of intense activity, both physical and mental, and an excellent superfood for convalesence after illness. Chicken, especially, is a versatile food that any child can enjoy.

chicken

Until the time of factory farming and intensive raising methods, chicken and turkey were luxury meats. Both are now so cheap that they are everyday foods, but the price we pay is a lack of flavour and texture, a higher saturated-fat content and the risk of chemical residues like antibiotics and growth-promoting hormones. It's much better to spend more on free-range organic poultry and eat a little less of it.

Chicken meat contains much less fat than red meats, and, since most of this is contained in the skin, it's easily removed. As well as protein, chicken provides easily absorbed iron and zinc – twice as much in the dark meat as in the breast. This makes it excellent food during pregnancy, and a blood- and resistance-builder for children of all ages.

Roast chicken should have all the fat removed from inside the body cavity. It should then be cooked on a roasting rack so that all the fat drips into the bottom of the pan. Don't cook potatoes in this fat: roast them in a separate dish drizzled with olive oil and sprinkled with rosemary. Enjoy the succulent flavor of chicken, but don't eat the skin.

A **rich source** of protein and most B vitamins, and a **good source** of iron and zinc.

wonderful chicken soup

All poultry can be used to make soup, though it is important to remove as much fat as possible from the stock, either by skimming or blotting it off, or by refrigerating overnight so the hardened fat can be removed in the morning.

The traditional Chicken Soup beloved of Jewish mothers has more than folklore to thank for its nickname, "Jewish penicillin." Researchers have found a special sulphur compound in chicken soup that really does protect against throat and chest infections. The protein content of soups made from chicken and other poultry is also very easily absorbed, which makes them perfect invalid food. It's possible that a poor immune system, chronic fatigue, and glandular fever may all be aggravated by poor protein absorption, particularly in the presence of digestive difficulties. Chicken soup could be the answer.

turkey

The modern farmed turkey is a pale and insipid descendant of its wild ancestor in North America. But if you can find a free-range organic bird, you will be well-rewarded. Unlike other poultry, turkey is extremely low in fat, containing only 2.7g per 3½oz/100g. It's rich in protein and supplies some well-absorbed iron and zinc, more in the dark meat than the white.

The low fat content tends to make it a dry insipid bird when cooked unless great care is taken. Generally speaking, the smaller the bird, the less it dries out and the better the flavor. Many children prefer delicious cold leftover turkey, which can also be used in curries and hashes.

A **rich source** of protein and vitamin B_{12}; a **good source** of other B vitamins, potassium, and zinc.

duck

Duck is rich in protein, minerals, and lots of the B vitamins. Delicious though the crispy skin is, you will get 29g of fat if you eat 4oz/125g of meat and skin, but only 9.7g if you just eat the meat. Always cook duck on a rack. Prick the skin all over with a sharp fork or skewer first, so the fat layer under the skin can trickle out and fall under the rack as it melts in the heat of the oven. Served with apple sauce, duck not only tastes wonderful, but benefits from the pectins in the apple which help the body eliminate much of the cholesterol from the duck.

With the huge popularity of Chinese food, many children get their first taste of duck served with plum sauce, scallions, cucumber, and buckwheat pancakes in the local Chinese restaurant. You couldn't have a healthier combination.

A **rich source** of protein, iron, zinc, potassium, and nearly all the B vitamins.

COOKING POULTRY SAFELY

The vast majority of our intensively reared chicken meat is infected with salmonella bacteria. While this does not present a health hazard when chicken is thoroughly and properly cooked, undercooked chicken is an extremely common cause of food poisoning.

- When cooking chicken and other poultry at home make sure that frozen birds are thoroughly defrosted – 24 hours in a refrigerator – before cooking.
- If roasting, make sure the oven is fully up to temperature before placing the bird inside.
- To check that poultry is cooked, prick the thickest part of the thigh with a fork or skewer to see that juices run clear.
- If barbecuing chicken, it's best to partially cook it first to guarantee that it is cooked right through when finished on the barbecue.
- Any poultry which is still pink when you cut it, or has juices that still appear bloodstained, should never be eaten.
- Observe the rules of kitchen hygiene when preparing, handling, and cooking poultry (see pages 114–15).

QUICK FOOD IDEA

A delicious pita filling from left-over cooked poultry. Dice the cold poultry into small cubes. Heat 1 tablespoon olive oil in a deep frying-pan. Add 1 crushed garlic clove, 3 finely chopped spring onions, with their green tops, and 1 medium potato, peeled and diced into small cubes. Cook gently for 5–6 minutes until soft. Add the poultry, increase the heat, and cook for 5 minutes, stirring frequently. Serve hot in warmed whole wheat pita breads.

super fish

Fish is an **outstanding superfood**. It is rich in **protein**, low in **fat**, and loaded with B vitamins and **precious minerals** from the seas which were the origin of all **life on earth**. Sea fish are particularly valuable for their **high iodine** content. The oily fish are important sources of vitamins A, D, and E and the omega-3 **essential fatty acids**.

at the fish counter

When buying **fresh fish** check that the eyes are bright and shiny, not dull or sunken in to the head, that the skin still has lots of scales, and that gills are still red. Fish should always have the fresh smell of the sea. Look for bright, clear spots on flounder and well-defined markings on other fish.

When buying **shellfish** check that they feel heavy for their size. All molluscs should be closed. All shellfish should be eaten on the day you buy it. Above all, buy your shellfish from a regular supplier whose reputation you can rely on.

Watch out for additives in **processed fish**. Colorings, preservatives, and flavorings are commonly used in the coating of fish fingers, and brown and yellow dyes on smoked haddock. Growing public concern about additives in recent years has meant that more manufacturers have given up using them and haddock is beginning to be widely available.

at home

All fish are particularly nutritious for children since they are easily digestible and quick to cook. Another bonus is that if you buy seasonally some can be extremely inexpensive. If your children already like fish sticks, it won't be too hard to persuade them to be just a bit more adventurous.

As a rule of thumb, all fish take 5 minutes per 1 inch/2.5 cm of thickness to cook, no matter how large the fish or whether it is baked, steamed, broiled or pan-fried.

• When baking, put the fish into a preheated oven. If cooking whole fish, score the surface with two or three deep cuts, brush with olive oil, and sprinkle with herbs and lemon juice.

• Steaming can also be done in the oven by wrapping the fish in a loose but tightly sealed foil parcel. For traditional steaming, an ideal and cheap utensil is the Chinese bamboo steamer, which works well and is easy to handle.

white fish

These are all very similar from a nutritional standpoint, whether sea fish like cod, haddock, whiting, monkfish, sea bream, catfish, red and grey mullet, snappers, flounder, sole, and halibut, or freshwater fish like pike, perch, bream, or carp. They contain virtually no fat, few calories, and plenty of the protein needed by young children.

They all contain the B vitamins but not much iron and although halibut (which is slightly oily), may contribute a little vitamin A, the white fish do not generally supply fat-soluble vitamins.

Cod and halibut livers are very rich in vitamins A, D, and E, but these aren't eaten, just used for the production of oil.

oily fish

Oily fish like mackerel, salmon, trout, tuna, herring, anchovies, sardines, whitebait and eel contain high levels of eicosapentanoeic acid, one of a group of fatty acids belonging to the omega-3 family. These are known to be essential to healthy cell function, especially in the brain, and their anti-inflammatory action can be extremely valuable in the relief of psoriasis and eczema.

When buying fish canned in oil take care to read the labels. Avoid those marked "vegetable oil" since this is certain to contain palm oil which is high in saturated fat. Choose instead fish canned in olive, sunflower, or safflower oil and drain off the surplus before serving it, or buy fish canned in water.

Oily fish are often smoked to preserve them and, though little of their nutritional value is lost, a great deal of salt is added before the smoking process. Eating large amounts of smoked food has been linked to a higher incidence of cancer, so smoked oily fish should be regarded as occasional treats.

shellfish

These can be divided conveniently into the crustaceans: crabs, lobsters, shrimp, and crayfish; and the molluscs: mussels, oysters, cockles, sea urchins, winkles, clams, and scallops. All shellfish contain the same amount of protein and other nutrients as white fish, though they are much saltier. The vitamin and mineral content of the crustaceans is the same as white fish. Molluscs contain much more iron and vitamin A and they are also good sources of zinc, especially oysters, which, together with cockles and snails, contain as much iron as a fillet steak. Snails are an even richer source of this essential mineral, supplying as much as the equivalent weight of meat or poultry liver.

HEALTH WARNING

Shellfish are a fairly common cause of severe food allergy reactions. If children have had one bad reaction, be extremely careful to make sure they avoid eating shellfish again (see page 204).

super dairy products

Dairy products are widely consumed in the Western world, where they are a key ingredient in many of the foods children enjoy most, such as ice cream, milkshakes, pizza, lasagne, and pasta dishes. They are a major source of bone-building calcium, essential for the healthy growth and development of all children.

milk

Milk is our very first food, and the COW'S milk so widely drunk in the Western world is great stuff for growing children. When in the 1930s undernourished Scottish schoolchildren were given a daily pint of milk, their growth rate accelerated approximately 20 percent, and there was an obvious improvement in health and vitality.

Milk provides bone-building calcium, plenty of protein, zinc for the immune system and growth generally, and some vital B vitamins, including folic acid and vitamin B_{12}. Because they graze in grassy fields, cows produce milk that is always a rich source of vitamins A, D, and E, and of a special fatty acid (CLA) which may help protect against a number of cancers, including melanoma (skin cancer) and leukemia. The vitamins A, D, and E are all found in cream, for which reason children under five should always be given whole milk, not skim or semi-skim.

Wonderful food that it can be, however, the milk news is not all good. Bones need magnesium as well as calcium, and other trace elements, all poorly supplied in milk. In many parts of the world, people lack the enzyme lactase needed for its digestion, and millions of people in the West are allergic or sensitive to it. Eczema, asthma, colic in babies, and hyperactive behavior have all been linked with milk, as have sinus and respiratory problems (see Allergies, page 204). In addition, a glass of milk contains nearly 5 g of saturated fat.

Children who cannot tolerate cow's milk may thrive on goat milk, available in most natural food stores and in some supermarkets. The various substitute "milks" on the market, particularly those based on SOY, are rich in protein, and some are fortified to provide extra calcium. But these soy drinks lack most of the B vitamins and other trace elements found in true milk. Some experts are questioning, too, the wisdom of giving small children regular doses of the isoflavones found in soy drinks.

Organic milk is now widely available. Free of the traces of antibiotics, growth hormones, and pesticides liable to lurk in ordinary milk, it is worth the extra cost hundreds of times over for your child's health.

cheese

Cheese is another great food for growing children – though with the possible problems of milk (see page 204). It is a food that adds a huge range of wonderful tastes and textures to the diet. The hard cow's-milk cheeses, such as Cheddar, tend to be the highest in fat, but they are also the highest in protein, in calcium – a 2oz/60g chunk of Cheddar will supply your day's calcium needs – and in zinc, which is needed by developing brains, skin, and the immune system and which could also help protect children from anorexia and other eating disorders.

Introduce children to a wide range of cheeses, including soft young goat cheeses (older goat cheeses become much sharper and develop a distinctive flavor that many people dislike), but save the blue cheeses until children are older. Cheeses made from sheep milk may be easier to digest: they include the wonderful Spanish Manchego – in Spain you can choose the degree of maturity and sweetness you prefer – and Greek feta cheese, which is hard, white, and crumbly and very good in salads.

QUICK FOOD IDEAS

The plowman's lunch – 2 or 3 different cheeses, whole wheat rolls, and coleslaw – could be a quick, tasty, and nutritious weekend lunch.

Granny Smith's Welsh Rarebit (see page 155).

Pizza-style Bread (see page 198).

Greek salad: diced cucumber, chunks of tomato and green bell pepper, onion rings, and black olives, dressed with olive oil, lemon juice, fresh herbs, and seasonings tossed with cubes of feta cheese.

cottage cheese

Most children love cottage cheese, a curd cheese that is low in fat, mild-tasting, and far easier to digest than ordinary cheese. And it has lots of protein. The Indian cheese, panir, is made from curd cheese pressed solid and cut into cubes. Cottage cheese is so mild that you can eat it with either savory or fruity accompaniments, and as such it can turn a snack into a nutritious meal. Cottage cheese is a must for the family refrigerator – but eat it within a few days of purchase since dried-out cottage cheese is not pleasant.

QUICK FOOD IDEAS

Supper for a hot day: cottage cheese with chunks of peach or nectarine, a few strawberries, or a handful of grapes.

Slices of tomato and cucumber tossed with cottage cheese, served on lettuce leaves with plenty of fresh basil, cilantro or parsley and a drizzle of extra-virgin olive oil.

yogurt

One of the fermented foods developed by primitive people the world over, yogurt is definitely in the superfood category, being rich in calcium, protein, and some important B vitamins. It is much more easily digested than milk for children or adults who are lactose intolerant (see page 204). And, importantly, it works wonders for the digestive system.

The human intestine is host to several billion bacteria. Most of them are good guests, helping protect us from less friendly bacteria, and new research suggests that they may also play a key role in the healthy functioning of the immune system. Occasionally these good guys get wiped out, either by pathogenic bacteria, or by a course of antibiotics..

All fresh yogurts, except those pasteurized for a longer shelf life, contain lactic acid bacteria, and may also contain varying amounts of others, such as bifidus. Look for yogurts that are listed as "live"; these yogurts contain extra quantities of useful bacteria. Sometimes available in natural food markets but difficult to find, you can buy live yogurt cultures and make your own from safe, unpasteurized milk. Yogurt makers are getting very serious about the health-giving properties of their product. Remember that the fresher yogurt is, the higher its bacterial content; remember, too, that pasteurized yogurts do not contain these bacteria and are no longer "live."

Flavored fruit yogurts almost always proclaim virtuously that they are low fat or fat-free. No doubt they hope this will distract attention from the sugar or sweeteners, coloring, flavoring, stabilizers, emulsifiers, and other chemical additives such yogurts usually contain. Since 3½oz/100g ordinary yogurt contains only a single gram of fat, don't be fooled. Buy thick natural yogurt – Greek yogurt is delicious; buy it for special occasions – and add your own fruit. Introduce children, too, to sheep milk yogurt – which they may like even more: and when they're very young, give them goat milk yogurt, even easier for them to digest.

QUICK FOOD IDEAS

Stir puréed fruit, or crushed strawberries and raspberries, or a spoonful of a no-sugar fruit spread into natural yogurt. Blend with fresh orange juice and water for a refreshing summer drink.

Stir fresh mint, grated cucumber, a little olive oil, salt, and a touch of lemon juice into natural live yogurt for a lovely summer salad.

eggs

One of the most important substances in egg yolk is lecithin, which is vital as part of many of the body's metabolic processes, including the dispersal of dangerous fat deposits and cholesterol. Lecithin helps to prevent the development of heart disease and the formation of gall stones and also encourages speedy conversion of body fats into energy. Because of their high lecithin content eggs are an important brain food, contributing not only to memory and concentration, but also to good mental and emotional status. Eggs are also rich in protein, zinc, vitamins A, D, E, and B_{12}.

How sad it is that the obsession with cholesterol has resulted in the humble egg being branded as a villain in the control of heart disease.

Another health concern has caused people to turn against eggs even more – the scare of the possibility of eggs containing the salmonella enteritidis bacteria. The risk of infection is far, far less in a well-run organic farm where the chickens are not crowded and have a large free-range area. The best protection is to buy only free-range organic eggs from a certified supplier. These eggs will provide one of the best nutritional values-for your money. However, it is not advisable for pregnant women, the very young or elderly, and anyone with compromised immune systems to eat raw or undercooked eggs.

While health experts advise no more than three or four eggs per week, the World Health Organisation advocates a total of 10, including those used in cooking. Eggs are an amazing source of high quality protein. Just two boiled eggs supplies a quarter of a day's need which, with their other nutrients, makes them a true superfood for children of all ages. Eggs in almost any form are the perfect quick food for children from older babies to teenagers. We suggest some ideas below.

HEALTH WARNING

Eggs are quite a common cause of allergy (see page 204) and some authorities believe that introducing eggs too early in a baby's diet can increase the risk of allergy. Between six and nine months is usual, but later rather than sooner is advisable if there is a history of allergy in your family. In some children asthma attacks can be triggered by eggs.

QUICK FOOD IDEAS

Eggy triangles: cut medium-thick bread into triangles. Heat 1 tablespoon vegetable oil in a frying pan. Beat 1 lightly seasoned egg until smooth and dip the bread triangles in it. Fry the triangles in the oil until golden on both sides. Drain on paper towels.

Flavored scrambled eggs: lightly cook chopped tomato in a little melted butter and pour scrambled-egg mixture over it. When the egg is almost done, sprinkle a little grated cheese on top.

Mix chopped hard-boiled egg with mayonnaise and chopped cucumber for a sandwich filling or open sandwich topping.

super fats

Without some fats meals would lose their savor and interest. And without the right fats, children cannot grow and think. Vegetable oils, for instance, provide the fats we need to hold our cells together, insulate us from the cold, supply energy, and deliver the important vitamins A, D, E, and K.

The whole question of fats is complicated and confusing, but understanding the different types of fats, what they do, how much we need, and how much is healthy, is a vital step on the path to nutritional good health (see page 16). All of the healthy fats and oils make a major contribution to the calorie consumption of small children. These calories come in abundance from small amounts of the fats and oils, so it is much easier for youngsters to get their calorie needs from these than from having to eat huge amounts of the bulky foods that would be needed for the equivalent calories.

It is now certain that the seeds of heart disease are sown in childhood, if not before, so getting your children into good habits regarding eating fats is vital to their long-term good health. Unsaturated fats, found mainly in vegetable oils like soy bean, corn, sunflower, and safflower and in oily fish, contain virtually as many calories as saturated fats, but they are extremely important for good health and should form a regular part of every child's daily diet.

HEALTH WARNING

Labels such as "cholesterol-free" or "low in cholesterol" on foods can be very misleading. It is the percentage of saturated fats that you have to look out for, avoiding foods high in them.

---

butter

Butter is delicious and when used in modest amounts is certainly better than any margarine, most varieties of which are high in unhealthy trans fats (see page 17). Butter is virtually all fat and 60 percent of that is saturated. But butter is also a rich source of vitamins A, D, and E so, used sparingly, it is useful for children. Unlike most dairy products, butter is a poor source of calcium and contains virtually no B vitamins.

vegetable oils

Oils provide enormous amounts of calories, 899 per 100g. Most vegetable oils contain little saturated fat and good supplies of vitamin E. Exceptions are palm oil and coconut oil, which both contain large amounts of saturated fat; also, coconut oil has virtually no vitamin E. Avoid buying packaged food if content label lists "vegetable oil"; it is likely to contain palm oil or coconut oil. Always buy named varieties of oil.

The polyunsaturated fats in vegetable oils are extremely important because they contain essential fatty acids that we do not make for ourselves.

When used in baking, oils retain most of their nutritional value, but when used for frying the percentage of polyunsaturated fats is reduced: up to 20 percent in quite a short cooking period.

Sunflower is the richest of vegetable oils in vitamin E. It and corn and safflower oils are ideal for light salad dressings and for cooking. Their light flavors may make them more acceptable to children than the richer olive oil.

Nut oils: walnut oil and hazelnut oil both contain important essential fatty acids, and gourmets love their strong and characteristic flavors, walnut especially, on green-leafed salads or added to boost the flavor of a stir-fry. These oils may be too strongly flavored for young palates, although teenagers may appreciate them.

Do not use nut oils if your child has nut allergies.

olive oil

Olive oil, enriched in monounsaturated fat, is a marvellous food-medicine. In traditional folk medicine, it has always been recommended as an enhancer of overall health and a remedy for digestive problems.

Recipes in this book specify "extra-virgin olive oil" for salads and dressings, but include "olive oil" for basic cooking such as stir-frying. Extra-virgin olive oil is expensive, but it is the healthiest

because the way in which the oil is extracted from olives does not lose any of its rich mineral, vitamin, essential fatty acid, and antioxidant content – or its wonderful flavor. Choosing the best possible olive oil – and cold-pressed varieties of other vegetable and nut oils, too – could help your children avoid a range of illnesses from arthritis and joint problems to heart disease and some forms of cancer.

cream and ice cream

OK, so *they are* high-fat, but cream and ice cream are among life's treats, so don't banish them from your home on that account: and as long as they are the healthy organic version – the only kind we'd give children – that fat is rich in sunshine

vitamins A, D, and E. Fromage frais or yogurt can often be substituted for cream – rich Greek yogurt from gourmet markets tastes great with a fruit salad – better than cream. And, of course, who would turn down ice cream on a hot day?

herbs & spices

Nearly every herb or spice commonly used in cooking has also been employed as a **medicine** down through the centuries. Almost all of them improve the digestion of foods to which you add them and most herbs and spices also have other **healing properties** that make them great additions to foods for young and old alike.

herbs

Parsley is rich in iron as well as antioxidants, beta-carotene, and chlorophyll, which make it great for tired, listless teenagers. It also contains good amounts of vitamin C. Add it to soups, salads, homemade vegetable juices, and sandwiches.

Sage is a great aid to the digestion of rich fatty foods: add a leaf to the pan when you fry sausages. It is also very effective against infections of the mouth and throat.

Rosemary enhances the memory, because it is a stimulant to the brain and to the nervous system. It is also a good general tonic. Add sprigs to a roast of spring lamb, or warm it in the olive oil in which cubed potatoes are to be baked.

Thyme is a powerful antiseptic and general tonic and has a good aromatic flavor – so it is a must in robust winter stews and casseroles.

Oregano gives pizzas their distinctive wonderful aroma and is also a powerful antiseptic (though it should not be used medicinally during pregnancy). Use it dried or fresh in tomato-based sauces, soups, and casseroles.

Basil is the perfect herb for children of all ages because it is calming and soothing – so it will be good for parents, too. The aromatic oils in fresh basil which produce these beneficial effects have an unmistakable aroma use in any tomato dish and all types of salads. It is an essential herb in pesto. Basil freezes well, but loses much of its aroma when dried.

Garlic offers protection for the heart, lungs, and digestive system and is also powerfully protective against all kinds of infection, so give your children plenty during winter months especially. Add it to soups, salads, and savory dishes – and kids love garlic bread.

Mint, the inseparable companion of new potatoes and roast lamb, has an uniquely soothing effect on the digestive system. Try peppermint tea for stomach upsets, too.

Chives are junior members of the great onion and garlic tribe, and add a fresh distinctive note to summer salads, especially cucumber and tomato.

Bay leaves, added to stocks and soups and to bean casseroles, help counter gas and wind. They are a natural aid to digestion.

Coriander is also very beneficial to the digestive process. Cilantro is the form of coriander which adds a wonderfully aromatic and tangy flavor to curries, rice dishes and salads.

spices

Chili peppers provide a boost to the circulation and are very helpful for the digestion. When cooking for children, try these fiery flavorings, whether fresh or dried, powdered or flaked, in tiny quantities at first.

Cinnamon warms the whole system, aiding circulation and digestion, and is powerfully antiviral, too. Use it in winter cakes, apple desserts, and hot drinks.

Cloves are another great winter warmer and antiseptic: use them in sauces, dried fruit compotes, and apple desserts.

Nutmeg is a warming aid to digestion. Grate it over winter vegetables like spinach, cabbage, and cauliflower just before you serve them.

Ginger turns up in almost every Chinese or Indian meat dish to improve its digestibility, protect against toxins, and improve flavor. Hot ginger tea will help ward off colds and chills, and children love crystallized ginger. Ginger is an effective remedy for nausea and travel sickness, so it is a good idea to have some crystallized ginger or a can of ginger ale handy when traveling with children.

Cumin is another digestive aid and nerve tonic, adding that unmistakably aromatic note to the kebabs and stews of Middle Eastern cooking. Don't keep ground cumin too long because it loses flavor quickly.

the danger foods

By the time your children are old enough to have reached the big wide world of the playground and the children's party circuit, you will have come to realize that much of the food their school friends eat most of the time is not exactly healthy. Foods once known as occasional treats have become part of our children's everyday eating.

According to recent research, as many as 99 percent of the food products advertised on television during children's viewing times is potentially unhealthy for them. And psychologist Dr Aric Sigman, who contributed to the research, pointed out that the advertisements "were crafted to exploit children's vulnerability at critical stages of their development."

There's nothing wrong with potato chips, French fries, cakes and chocolate when they are occasional treats. But the key word is occasional, and they will stop even being treats when children can have them any time they want. Explain to your children exactly why you're being selective – or, as they will probably see it, mean – with their treats. When they are big enough, show them how to read food labels and identify the cosmetic additives and the artfully disguised sugars. Teach them to be questioning about the endless parade of TV commercials aimed directly at them. Gently, little by little, instill into them a sound knowledge of nutrition. Show them how to make healthy choices.

One day your children will thank you; for the time being, you'd better get used to being unpopular quite often. But you know it is worth it.

On these pages is a run-down of the danger foods and drinks that you need to think twice about before giving them to your children.

caffeine

Tea and coffee are not drinks for small children. The caffeine in them renders them powerful stimulants which can easily make children edgy and hyperactive. The tannins in tea can interfere with the uptake of vital nutrients, including iron and magnesium. Keep children off both until they're at least six or seven; then, if they ask for it, give them tea in the form of a little milk mixed with hot water with just a small amount of tea. Green tea would be even better, but if you're drinking Indian tea yourself, don't expect children to choose green. There's caffeine in many of the most popular soft drinks, too: read the labels carefully so that you know what to avoid.

hamburgers

The hamburgers served in popular chain-restaurants or sold from the supermarket freezer section are likely to be made from the cheapest source of factory-farmed meat, with a high content of saturated fat and probably some chemical additives – color, preservatives, flavorings – thrown in for good measure. Meeting the gang for hamburgers at the local hamburger-bar is one of those teenage rites of passage that you would be highly unwise to forbid. But otherwise, either buy hamburgers from a trustworthy butcher, or make your own from good lean meat, or from grains and vegetables. There are plenty of recipes in Satisfying Suppers (see pages 164–187).

soft drinks

These drinks all have one thing in common: sweetness. Unless the drink is a 100 percent fruit juice, its sweetness will be provided by either sugar or artificial sweeteners. As well as these, carbonated drinks are also likely to contain flavorings, colors, and preservatives (see Additives, overleaf), carbon dioxide to provide the fizz, and phosphoric acid which can leach calcium out of bones and teeth. New research from Germany has also linked a high intake of phosphate-containing drinks with hyperactivity and other behavior problems. Seventy percent of carbonated drinks contain caffeine, which can quickly cause children who drink them to become addicted to caffeine.

Juice-based drinks, fruit sodas, and -ades can look like a more healthy choice than other soft drinks. But look at the label: in many of them, the fruit content is actually tiny and color, flavor, and preservatives may all be supplied by additives. Even pure fruit juices are not the best choice for children if they are drunk in quantity, because the fruit acids they contain can damage tooth enamel, while the natural sugars in fruit are still sugars and you can have too much of them.

So if you give your children fruit juice, serve it undiluted only on very special occasions, such as Sunday morning breakfast with all the family; otherwise, dilute it at least half and half with water. When you're really thirsty, there's nothing like water.

sugar

Sugar turns up in the most surprising foods: there is quite a lot of it in a can of baked beans, a jar of peanut butter, a readymade pasta sauce, and even potato chips. Food manufacturers love sugar because it is cheap, is an excellent preservative, and can help improve texture. In the US, Canada, Australia, and the UK, consumption of sugar is rising inexorably – not so much spooned out of the sugar-bowl at home as hidden in many foods and snacks eaten from babyhood onward. Sometimes, it is called sugar on the label. More often you'll find it lurking under its other names – sucrose, maltose, dextrose, dextrin, glucose, or invert sugar which sounds somehow harmless. They're all sugars and your children don't need them in these quantities. See Carbohydrates (page 13) to remind yourself why.

artificial sweeteners

There have been many question marks over the safety of the artificial sweeteners saccharin and cyclamates. So most manufacturers now go for aspartame, the brand-name of which is NutraSweet. If your children eat flavored yogurts, breakfast cereals, frozen desserts, refrigerated desserts or fruit spreads, if they drink any kind of soft drink including flavored milk, or if they chew gum, they could be ingesting NutraSweet. It may also be added to foods and drinks as well as sugar: it is much cheaper. But the scientific history of this popular sweetener is not reassuring.

Regular intake of aspartame has been linked to headaches, brain tumors, seizure (as in epilepsy), and mood disorders. The manufacturer of NutraSweet claims that there is "overwhelming scientific evidence" for its safety. In fact, of 166 studies into the safety of aspartame on human health, 74 had industry-related funding and all 74 gave it a clean bill; the remaining 92 were independently funded and only 12 failed to note some kind of adverse reaction.

However, a three-year study done at King's College, London, showed that the sweetener is not carcinogenic and carries no risk of brain tumors.

Other studies suggest that artificial sweeteners trigger sensations of hunger in the brain that lead to over-eating and, therefore, obesity.

additives

Back in the 1960s, thousands of impossibly hyperactive children became controllable and near-normal when they were put on a dict which excluded numbers of additives commonly used in food, particularly colorings such as (tartrazine). Some of these additives are no longer permitted in food eaten by children, but many still are, numbers of which have been linked to health problems such as asthma and eczema in vulnerable children, or those with behavioral disorders such as hyperactivity (see page 206), despite having passed safety tests. What has not yet been tested properly is how damaging they can be in the endless combinations in which they are consumed – and, in the case of children, in the quantities. Most additives, most of the time, are used to give eye or taste appeal, or longer shelf life, to high-fat/high-sugar or high-salt foods that are not particularly healthy anyway. Yogurts aimed at children are likely to be specially high in sugar and in additives. If in doubt about tartrazine, check in a good source (see Books to Read, page 216).

chocolate & candy

To a child a bar of chocolate is a gift-wrapped chunk of sheer deliciousness. To the detached eye, it is a lot of unhealthy hardened fat, sugar, chemical additives, and some cocoa solids. Most sweets are made to the same unhealthy recipe, only more so. European dark chocolate, especially the excellent organic versions, with at least 70 percent cocoa fat solids is a better choice than most children's bars. But it has a slightly bitter flavor, and is unlikely to appeal to young children. You will have to work out a strategy for limiting consumption of candy and chocolate that doesn't turn them into highly desirable foods, with all the extra appeal because they are something "forbidden."

cookies & cakes

Almost any homemade cookie or cake you can produce is going to taste better than the boring kinds on supermarket shelves – mixes of highly refined flour, sugar, hardened fats, and flavorings.

potato chips

Potato chips are a delicious crunchy treat. But an occasional treat is what they should remain. Why? First, they are more than one-third fat – even "low-fat" potato chips contain than 20 percent fat – and an unhealthy highly saturated fat at that, which will help clog up young arteries. Secondly, they contain a staggering amount of salt – over 1 gram in an average packet. Thirdly, they often contain sugar and, if they are "flavored," they will contain artificial flavorings, too.

ice cream

Proper ice cream made with cream, sugar, and perhaps fruit is delicious. It's pretty fattening stuff, but at least it can be said to be real food in most respects. Perhaps your best policy here is to serve real ice cream as part of a family meal for a treat and to hope to persuade your children into spurning the ghastly stuff available commercially. Read the labels on them: hydrated fats, lots of sugar, air, water, powdered milk, and plenty of chemical additives, and that's about it.

breakfast cereals

We have been brainwashed into seeing the average breakfast cereal as a nourishing, nutrient-packed food to give our children a great start to the day. Most cereals are far from this in reality: they have huge amounts of sugar by one or other of its names, a surprising amount of salt, and they're based on highly refined grains. A few cheap extra vitamins added will not compensate for such unhealthy eating. For plenty of better choices, see Big Breakfasts (pages 120–127).

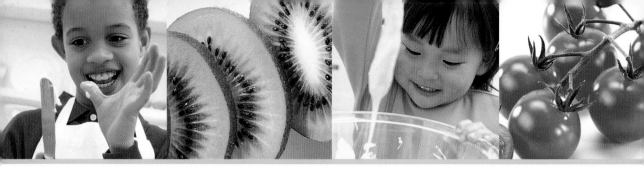

meals for every age group

As children grow, so their nutritional needs develop. Here, the essential foods for each childhood stage, from babyhood to the teenage years, are profiled and danger foods noted. Menu plans offer great ideas for feeding children super meals every day.

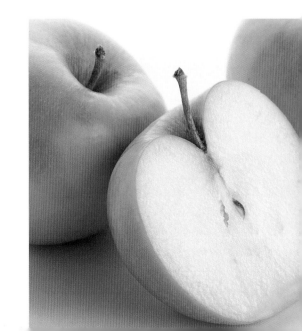

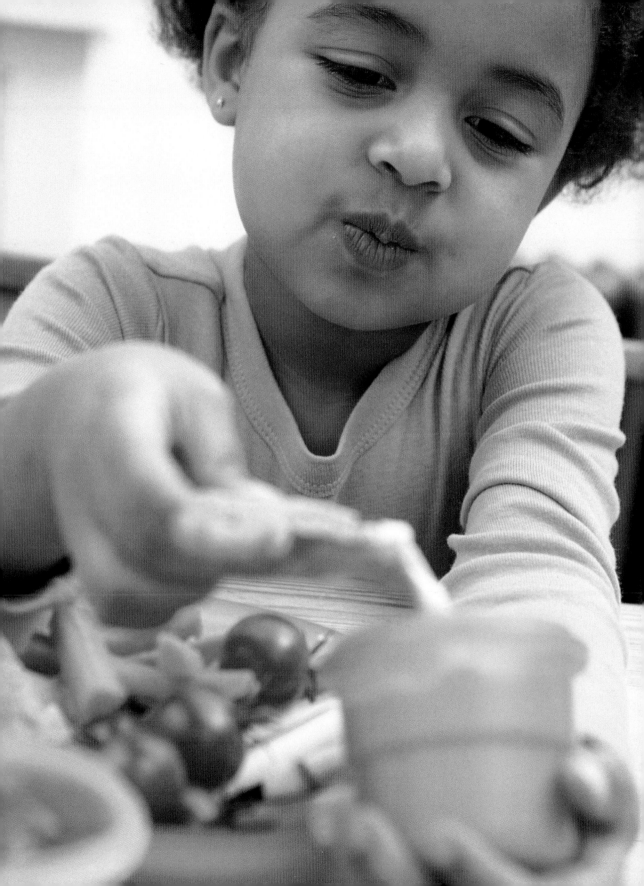

enjoying good food

Feeding children a generation or so ago was simpler than it is today. Mothers prepared purées for babies, more varied food for toddlers, and, after that, children ate with the family. Ice cream, sweets, chocolate, and potato chips were treats, not everyday fare, and there wasn't a hamburger chain at every intersection.

Today, the feeding of our children has become a heavily mined battlefield in which policies have to be carefully thought out and pursued, painful decisions made, and clever strategies devised. For the first two or three years, your children's diet is in your care. After that – from the first small toddlers' party for nursery-school friends – the world of commercial food marketing comes flooding in, and you will be up against it.

You will be up against your toddler's friends whose mothers allow them sweets, cookies, soft drinks, and potato chips every day. You will be up against the irresistible lure of that children's Mecca which seems so grown-up to them, the local hamburger joint. You will be up against an endless bombardment of commercials on the television shows your children watch, plugging junk food in every shape or form. You may be up against their school's unenlightened views on food service, the soft-drinks machine in the corridor and the hamburger-and-French fries van on the playground. And finally, you'll be up against the urge of all children to conform, not to be "different."

You will need to be firm. You'll have to say no much more often than you'd like. And you'll be treading a narrow path between a hard line which turns junk food into irresistible forbidden fruit, and the soft option of over-indulgence. It will undoubtedly be very, very tough. But you will be rewarded by healthy, vibrant children who are full of energy, with minds as active as their young bodies. You'll be rewarded by their growing realization of how much good health depends on what and how we eat. And you'll be rewarded by their enjoyment of authentically good food.

one stage at a time

In the following pages you'll find advice and tactics to deal with the problems and sort out the situations which may arise at the key stages of a child's development. There is also a special section for vegetarian children.

For each stage, there is listed half-a-dozen Superfoods especially appropriate for those years. And there are menu plans for Mondays to Fridays, for winter and summer, making great use of the recipes in this book. Since so many children pack a lunch for school, the menus feature suggestions for every weekday as well as ideas for simple lunches during vacations or holidays. For more ideas, see Tasty Lunches.

Weekends should be a break from routine for everyone, when schedules tend to go out of the window and pre-planned menus are inappropriate. But, hopefully, weekend eating will feature at least one relaxed family meal, when the children may be joined by their own friends, and for which you'll find plenty of ideas in the Recipes section.

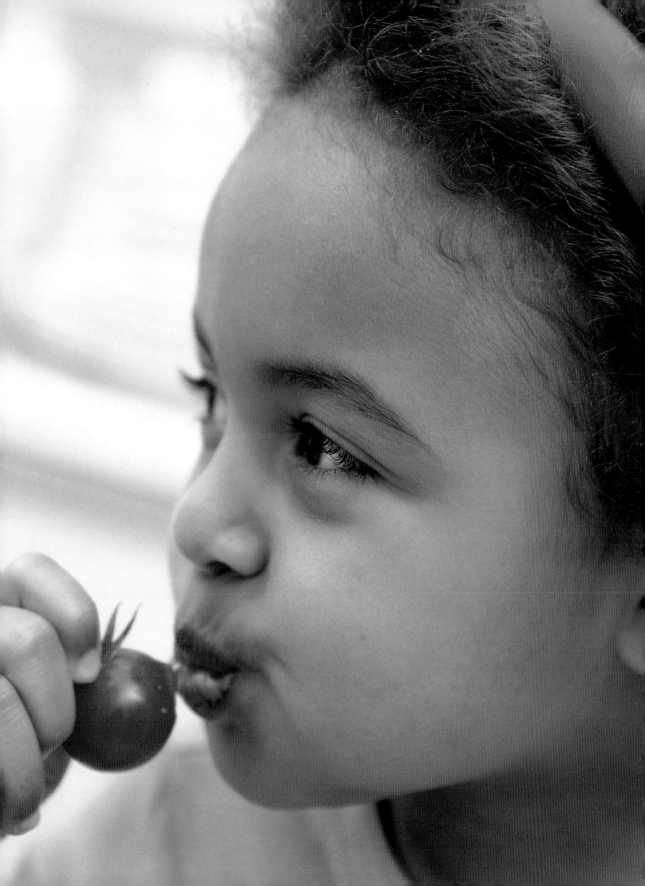

healthy babies from day one

There is no better time than when planning to have a baby for prospective parents to take a close look at their **lifestyles** and **eating habits**. For **healthy sperm,** viable eggs, and high fertility, optimum nutrition is needed and that means plenty of foods rich in **beta-carotene,** **folic acid**, **vitamin E**, **zinc**, **protein**, **B vitamins**, and **iron**.

Both alcohol and caffeine are known to damage sperm and these should be kept to a minimum for three months before planned conception. Nicotine is harmful to sperm (sperm counts have declined by 50 percent in the past 30 years) and also to developing babies so both prospective parents should quit smoking. But most importantly, you should both be eating as wide a variety of healthy, nutrient-packed foods as possible. This fact is emphasized by another alarming statistic: almost half the women attending fertility clinics have been on some form of restrictive weight-loss diet in the previous 12 months – a sure sign that what you eat plays a major role in fertility

food for mothers-to-be & the growing baby

Many experts advise a total ban on alcohol during pregnancy; others believe that two glasses of red wine a week will not do you or the baby any harm. Large amounts of caffeine should be avoided, since this substance can interfere with the absorption of iron and zinc from food.

Do not eat liver or liver pâté since they contain large amounts of vitamin A, too much of which can cause birth defects. Avoid unpasteurized milk or cheese, and any soft or blue cheeses, as they may contain the listeria which can be hazardous to the baby.

All red meats, including hamburgers, must be cooked thoroughly until there are no traces of pink; otherwise, there is a risk of E.coli infection. Poultry must be cooked until the juices run clear and there is no trace of pink in the meat; eggs should be cooked until the yolk is hard to protect against salmonella. Wherever possible, this really is the time to choose organic foods to avoid unwanted antibiotics, neurotoxic chemicals, and growth hormones.

Raspberry-leaf tea has been used by women for centuries as a tonic for the reproductive system. It should only be taken regularly in the last six weeks of pregnancy, when it will help to strengthen the long muscles of the uterus and assist with contractions and labor pains during labor.

pre-conception fitness for men

This pre-conception plan for men, to be started three months before trying for a baby, may sound cold and calculating, but it will dramatically increase the health and fertility of sperm, as well as being good for general fitness.

Stop smoking. There is growing evidence that cigarettes can reduce the level of male hormones, interfere with sperm development, and even cause congenital defects in babies.

Stop drinking alcohol, or at least drastically reduce your intake. Alcohol can severely damage sperm, so make sure you have no more than two or three drinks a week in the three months leading up to conception.

Watch your weight. Obesity interferes with hormone balance and may cause infertility.

Take 500mg **vitamin C** daily to reduce the risk of sperm clumping together in bunches. One month before you start trying for a baby, increase your intake to 1 gram a day.

Make sure you are eating **plenty of fruit,** especially oranges, kiwis, and orange and dark green fruit and vegetables.

Boost your intake of **zinc,** a mineral essential for reproduction, by adding lots of shellfish, particularly oysters, and pumpkin seeds to your diet.

Now is the time to stop high-caffeine **coffee** and **soft** drinks; weak Indian or green tea is all right in small amounts.

It is now essential to try to eat only **organic meat** to avoid the risk of added hormones.

eating healthily while pregnant

You are what you eat, and your baby is what you eat too, so ignore the friends, mother-in-law, grandmothers, or others who keep reminding you that you are "eating for two." You are not. You are eating for one and nourishing yourself and another.

Take care of yourself and your diet because you will have extra nutritional needs. At the same time, don't become a food freak, or obsessed by dieting

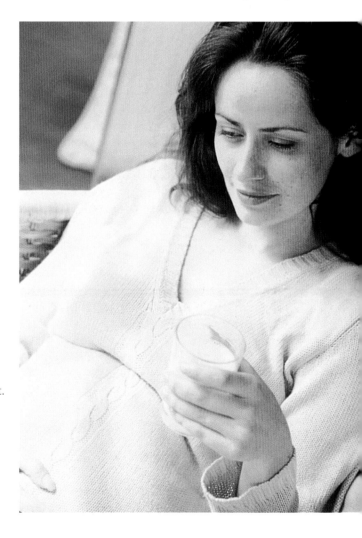

and don't worry about every bite you take. What you need is a simple common sense approach that will make sure you have a healthy pregnancy, a healthy baby, and the energy to look after it once it is born. This will also make sure you get back to your pre-pregnancy weight with as little effort as possible, though this will take longer – and, indeed, should not be a priority – if you are breast-feeding because you will need plenty of extra calories.

There is another "don't" that may seem obvious but very important: don't diet to lose weight unless you are advised to by your doctor. Instead, do some extra exercise, as long as there is no medical reason why you should not.

Many women have problems with digestion during the last month or so of pregnancy, because the bulge gets in the way. It is more comfortable to eat smaller amounts more often, making sure that your total food intake does not go up.

six superfoods for men and women

Shrimp High in protein and a good source of zinc, calcium, and iron, these are a delicious treat, but make the most of their low fat content by boiling or broiling – don't deep-fry them.

Fish A great source of vitamins A, B, and D, fish also supplies plenty of iodine, selenium, phosphorus, potassium, iron, and calcium. Most important during pregnancy, oily fish are a rich source of the essential fatty acids needed for the baby's developing brain. Choose fish that are low in mercury and PCBs; herring are better than farm-raised salmon.

Brown rice Eat this for its B vitamins, potassium, iron, protein, and fiber.

Broccoli A rich source of vitamins A and C, along with potassium and folic acid.

Citrus fruit These, and kiwis, are all super-rich in vitamin C; citrus fruit also provide important bioflavonoids to maintain the health of the circulatory system.

Natural yogurt Important for the extra calcium you need, yogurt also has all the beneficial probiotic bacteria which will keep your digestive system working efficiently so that you absorb maximum nutrients from your food. The bacteria also play an important part in stimulating your immune system, thus helping to protect against viral and bacterial infections.

eating plan for mothers-to-be

As a mother-to-be, you need a minimum of 2,200 calories a day – more if you are physically active – and it is important that you get these calories from a wide range of foods. Your total food intake should increase by around 20 percent, but your body's need for folic acid, vitamins B and C, calcium, zinc, and magnesium go up by far more.

Vegetarians, and particularly vegans, may be at risk of vitamin B_{12} deficiency and any woman who has been trying to lose weight by drastic dieting could be missing out on essential nutrients. If you are in either of these groups talk to your doctor about a vitamin and mineral supplement.

Eat lots of fresh fruit, vegetables, and salads. Try to stick to whole wheat cereals. During pregnancy food passes through your intestines more slowly to make sure that your body can absorb all the nutrients in it in order to nourish the baby. Consequently, constipation is common, so drink lots of water to prevent it.

sources of particular nutrients

You should be getting around 2oz (60g) of **protein** a day. A chicken leg has about 1oz (30g) protein, 1oz (30g) cheese has about ¼oz (7g), 6oz (180g) cod just over 1oz (35g), a two-egg omelette ½oz (15g), and 4oz (125g) cooked lentils just over ½oz (19g).

Canned sardines with the bones, low fat milk, yogurt, and cheese, beans, cereals, and nuts all provide extra **calcium,** and **essential fatty acids** are a bonus from the sardines.

Meat, chickpeas, leafy green vegetables, dried apricots, dates, and raisins will give you extra **iron** and **folic acid.**

Carrots, spinach, oily fish, eggs, dairy products, and dark green, orange, and yellow vegetables all provide **vitamin A** in safe amounts.

Green peppers, citrus fruit, kiwis, and most vegetables, including potatoes, contain **vitamin C** and **bioflavonoids. Vitamin D** is found in oily fish, eggs, and fish-liver oil, but it is also made by your body when you are out in the sunlight.

putting on weight

Weight gain during pregnancy is an important determinant of health for both mother and baby. The rate at which you gain weight varies during the nine months, with very little change occurring during the first 10 weeks. The healthy average during the second 10–12 weeks is about half a pound (250g) a week, and from then on or about one pound a week (500g).

If you think you are gaining too much weight during your pregnancy, do not put yourself on any form of restricted diet. Instead, ask for advice from your doctor. As a mother-to-be, you need a minimum of 2,200 calories a day – more if you are physically active – and it is important that you get them from a good mixture of different foods.

breast-feeding & baby meals

The best possible start in life you can give your baby is breast-feeding. There is now overwhelming evidence that formula milks, even those based on the latest nutritional findings, can never rival mothers' milk – the perfect first food for babies.

Research carried out with premature babies, and published in the *British Medical Journal* in November 1998, suggests that nutrition during the earliest weeks of a baby's life has a critical impact on brain development as well as on general health in later life. Vital fats known as long-chain polyunsaturated fatty acids, including DHA and AA, present in mothers' milk but not routinely added to commercial formula, may be one reason for this.

Breast-feeding also helps babies develop stronger immune systems. Numbers of studies, in developed and developing countries, show that breast-fed babies have higher resistance to childhood infections, are less likely to become anemic, and – if breast-feeding is continued until they are at least four months old – are much less likely to develop those modern diseases of childhood, asthma and eczema. It might be years before scientists succeed in identifying all the complex protective substances in mothers' milk: a recent discovery was lactoferrin, present in colostrum, the first and richest breast milk, which supplies powerful immune-boosting factors for the newborn baby.

Babies who are breast-fed may also be less likely to grow up into overweight children: a study of 9,000 Bavarian children, published in the *British Medical Journal* in July 1999, found that more bottle-fed babies had grown up into obese children than breast-fed babies. However, this protective effect was linked to the length of time the babies had been breast-fed and applies only to babies who have been breast-fed six months or longer.

There are other good reasons for breast-feeding. It is simpler than bottle-feeding; the milk does not need to be warmed in specially sterilized bottles and is always there in just the right quantities; and, most importantly, breast-feeding establishes an unique bond between mother and baby.

organic eating and mothers' milk

Sadly, for all its wonderful advantages, mothers' milk today is known to be contaminated with a number of pesticide residues and other toxic substances that no one is happy to see in babies' food. Dioxins, toxic chemicals called PCBs, and traces of persistent pesticides such as DDT and lindane have all been found in human breast-milk at worrying levels, although they are seldom found in formulas. However, a comprehensive Dutch study in the mid-1990s could detect no negative effects of this exposure in breast-fed infants with measurable body-levels of these pollutants. And the positive advantages of breast-feeding were still present. While this means that the message is still that feeding from the breast is best, it also means that breast-feeding mothers should eat 100 percent organic if they possibly can.

Many of the problems that new mothers experience with breast-feeding can be resolved with a little expert help. Even if breast-feeding proves too difficult at birth and the mother chooses to bottle-feed, it is often possible to re-establish breast-feeding, with the help of a trained breast-feeding counselor (see Resources, page 214).

But if the difficulties are insuperable, make sure you are giving your baby the best possible formula milk (see Resources, page 214).

foods to avoid while breast-feeding

When you are breast-feeding, much of what you eat or drink yourself is going to reach your baby through your milk. So if you or your partner have a family history of allergic problems such as hay fever or asthma, it would be a good idea to restrict your intake of or, if possible, omit altogether such well-known allergy-triggers as wheat and dairy products (see page 204). In a recent Scandinavian study of breast-fed babies suffering from colic, almost all the incidents of colic disappeared when their mothers stopped eating dairy products.

Highly spiced, chili-laden "hot" foods such as curries and "Tex-Mex" food, lots of tea and coffee, and alcohol in large quantities are other substances that could make your baby uncomfortable – or, in the case of caffeine, even keep him awake. Strong-tasting foods like onions and garlic may affect the taste of breast-milk and are perhaps best eaten in moderation by mothers while they are breast-feeding their babies.

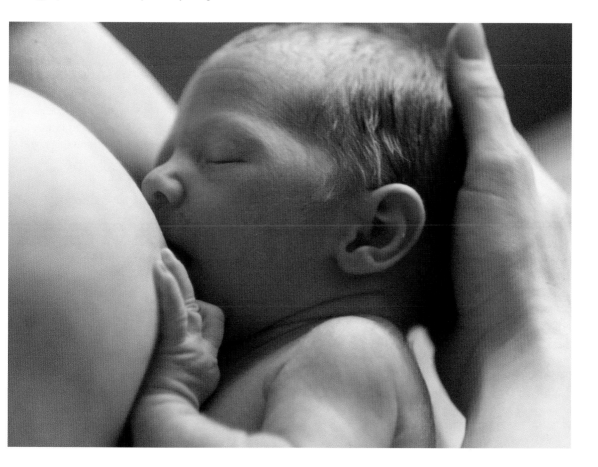

baby meals from 4-12 months

Whether your baby is breast-fed or bottle-fed, by the time he's around four months old, he is probably ready to start experimenting with solid foods. Let him make the choice. If he drops off to sleep soon after breast or bottle and sleeps peacefully till the next feeding, starting him on solid food can wait.

If, however, he's acting hungry long before feeding time, if he's still asking for more when the breast- or bottle-feeding is over, it is time to start trying him on something more substantial – but only after his milk feeding. Try introducing some little tastes in a small soft plastic baby-feeding spoon from time to time. Little purées of fruit and vegetables are a good start. If he pushes them away after just a taste or so, don't persist. Give it a rest for a few days then try again. And remember that he's still getting all the nourishment he needs at this stage from breast or bottle.

But if he's hungry for more, give it to him. By the time your baby has been taking purées for two or three months, he will be quite used to eating and will be learning to chew or even bite with his gums even if he doesn't have a single tooth. Now it is time to ease off the blender-made purées and start giving him food with more chewiness and texture to it: what the baby–food companies usually call Junior Foods. Food you prepare for him can now be mashed with a fork instead of blended, and you can actually cook the same meal for yourself and your baby, but remember not to salt and pepper the food during cooking and not to season the portion you give him.

It is in these early months of solid food that feeding problems may show up. Babies tend to pick mealtimes as a good moment to assert their independence. Pushing away food lovingly prepared for them is one great way to do this. (It may also mean, of course, that they are "just not hungry now, thank you.") Showing disappointment, frustration, or anger is playing their game. The more you insist, the more their mouths will stay provokingly shut. Remain smilingly unmoved. After a little while, remove the rejected food. And don't replace it.

superfoods for babies

Broccoli should be steamed or cooked in just a little water until it is soft enough to mash and strain. It is a good first food, but may be a little strong-tasting on its own, so try mixing it with strained boiled potato or baby rice.

Turnip, like broccoli, should be steamed or cooked in just a little water until it is soft enough to mash or strain. Along with other root vegetables, it blends well and is a good first food.

Avocado should be soft and ripe. Just mash it a little with a fork, or mix to a purée with breast or formula milk.

Carrots are a sweet and nutritious first food. As with broccoli and turnip, they can be steamed, or cooked in a little water until they are soft enough to purée.

Spinach can be a teaspoonful from a package of frozen chopped spinach, thawed and served at room temperature. Add it to a baby's diet from about six months old.

White fish is another nutritious food to add to a baby's diet from about six months. Give a tiny scoop of cod, flounder, or hake, making sure it has absolutely no bones in it.

the eating plan

Babies are receptive to a wide range of tastes, including broccoli, cabbage, and mild curry, between the ages of four and six months, when foods need to be puréed to a smooth and quite liquid consistency. Even when their initial reaction is a pained or surprised look, a second or third taste of the food is often accepted.

This "window" of developing taste-buds is brief, however, lasting no more than seven to eight weeks. By the time they are seven months old, most babies have developed strong preferences or dislikes, and babies this age are likely to spit out any novel food. If the only tastes a baby has known while the "window" is still open are the bland sweet pap of most commercial baby foods, you'll have your work cut out for years to make him eat from a wide and nourishing range of foods.

For this reason, we have chosen the Superfoods (listed in overleaf) from the sharp end of the taste palate. Other foods you can be giving your baby from about six months are any fruit soft and ripe enough to be mashed, hard-boiled eggs, and any vegetable tender enough to mash when it is cooked. You could offer a spoonful of hummus – make sure it is unsalted – a little poached salmon or chicken, or some baked apple with a touch of ground cinnamon or nutmeg. You can introduce dairy foods like yogurt or cottage cheese, or stir grated cheese into soups or vegetables. You can offer the first cereals now, such as oatmeal soaked overnight in breast or formula milk, creamy rice, and cooked millet cereal. And after six months – but no sooner – try him on wheat-based cereals (see Big Breakfasts, pages 120–127, for recipes).

When you introduce a new food, let two or three days go by before trying another; if digestive problems occur, you will know the likely cause.

By the age of 9–12 months your baby will have a few teeth and some very strong views on what he's prepared to eat. He should still be getting the same amount of either breast milk or formula, but he'll be ready for three meals a day, with milk as his regular drink. He'll be cutting teeth and needing hard chewy foods to help him learn to bite: give him strips of whole wheat toast baked in the oven, strips of carrot, crisp apple, or young turnip, and florets of broccoli or cauliflower. And he'll be ready for more sophisticated tastes, such as soups and stews made aromatic with herbs, puréed fish, a taste of your favorite pasta, savory rice, a few forkfuls of roast lamb, garlicky roasted vegetables with couscous, and cauliflower or broccoli cheese. Try to keep the menu as varied as possible (see overleaf).

foods to avoid

Any of the Danger Foods on pages 66–69 are inappropriate for babies. Some are especially perilous. Avoid sugar in any form other than the natural sugars present in fruit and vegetables – or your baby could be stuck with a sweet tooth for life. Avoid salt even when cooking vegetables, soups, or other dishes you couldn't imagine eating unsalted: salt can actually be a killer for babies.

Studies have also shown that babies are far more at risk than adults from pesticide residues, and that cancer and damaged immune and nervous systems may result from regular exposure. This is why organic foods (see pages 22–23) are so important for babies.

Avoid nuts in any shape or form: nut allergies are becoming tragically common.

Be sparing with fruit juices. Their concentrated sugars make them undesirable unless they are diluted at least half and half with water. And water is something your baby should be developing a taste for, too, by this time.

Those little jars and cans of commercial baby-food can be life-saving for busy mothers; as far as possible, stick to the organic brands, and check that they are not padded out with cheap low-nutrient fillers such as modified starch. And make sure they contain *no added sugars* of any kind. For excellent brand-names see Resources, page 214.

menus for a 6-month-old baby

sunday

10am: Apple and Apricot Purée (see page 124), with a little yogurt.

2pm: Root Vegetable and Potato Purée (see page 136). Peeled and grated ripe pear.

6pm: Potato mashed with a little cottage cheese. Mashed banana.

monday

10am: The yolk of a hard-boiled egg with strips of crustless whole wheat bread soaked in milk.

2pm: Turnip and carrot purée. Grated apple with a little orange juice.

6pm: Stewed apricots blended with yogurt.

tuesday

10am: Banana Cereal (see page 120).

2pm: Spinach purée with cottage cheese. A little mashed banana.

6pm: Carrot, broccoli, and potato purée.

wednesday

10am: Banana mashed with a little yogurt and wheatgerm.

2pm: Roast Chicken Puréed with Vegetables (see page 167). Mashed fresh pear.

6pm: Millet muesli (see page 48) with a little mashed peach or nectarine.

thursday

10am: Muesli (see page 120).

2pm: Root Vegetable and Potato Purée (see page 136). Peeled and grated ripe peach.

6pm: Stewed apple with yogurt. Strips of whole wheat bread soaked in milk.

friday

10am: Banana mashed with yogurt and a little wheatgerm.

2pm: Broccoli, Green Bean, and Sweet Potato Purée (see page 136). Puréed avocado with a few drops of lemon juice.

6pm: Muesli (see page 120) with a little grated fresh apple.

saturday

10am: Yolk of hard-boiled egg with whole wheat toasts.

2pm: Fishy Feast (see page 139). Turnip and carrot purée.

6pm: Mashed banana with orange juice.

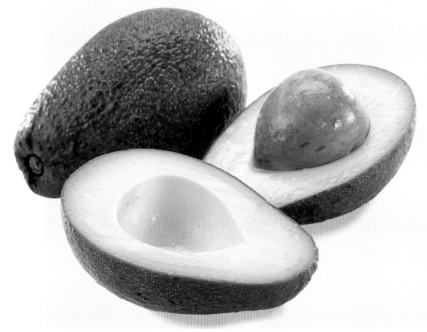

menus for an 18-month-old baby

sunday

breakfast: Scrambled egg with strips of whole wheat bread and butter.

lunch: Cold roast chicken (see page 167) with braised carrots, new potatoes and broccoli. Strips of fresh peach.

dinner: Baked potato mashed with cottage cheese and spinach purée. Fresh apple.

monday

breakfast: Muesli with yogurt and grated apple.

lunch: Egg and Spinach Mornay (see page 198). Fresh fruit salad.

dinner: Baked apple stuffed with raisins. Strips of buttered whole wheat toast and sliced cheese.

tuesday

breakfast: Banana Cereal (see page 120).

lunch: Haddock Moussaka (see page 164) with puréed broccoli. Strips of fresh pineapple.

dinner: Beanburger (see page 184) with mashed potatoes. Strips of celery and carrot.

wednesday

breakfast: Dried prunes and apricots soaked overnight, blended with a little yogurt.

lunch: Tomato and Cheese Bread Pudding (see page 143) with puréed spinach.

dinner: Split Pea and Rice Soup (see page 134). Strips of whole wheat toast and butter. Sticks of carrot.

thursday

breakfast: Muesli (see page 120) with yogurt and a sliced peach or pear.

lunch: Poached Chicken (see page 166). Steamed broccoli with a little butter and nutmeg. A peach.

dinner: Minestrone with Rice and Tomatoes (see page 130). Oatcakes with a little cheese (see page 158)

friday

breakfast: Fruit salad of kiwis, apple, and grapes, with Greek yogurt.

lunch: Riceburger (see page 183) with peas. A banana.

dinner: Sticks of celery and carrot with cottage cheese. Apple crumble.

saturday

breakfast: Whole wheat cereal with goats milk and raisins.

lunch: A baked potato with Roasted Vegetables (see page 174) with chopped tomato and cucumber salad.

dinner: Irish Stew (see page 168). Apple purée with Greek yogurt.

hungry toddlers

Your baby is now a toddler with a mind of his own, amazing energy, and a need to explore and to test his world. In order to fuel all that activity, he needs plenty of good carbohydrates which are found in grains like wheat, rice, and oats; in legumes like beans and lentils; in starchy vegetables such as carrots and potatoes; and in fruit and milk.

Since this is also a period of active growth, toddlers need high-quality protein, too. But remember that this doesn't mean only meat, fish, and eggs. Grains also contribute protein to the diet, and some grains are richer in protein than others: oats, millet, and amaranth, an ancient, newly revived grain, for instance (see page 51). Remember, too, that wholegrains are significantly higher in protein than those refined to produce white flour and white rice.

Once toddlers are eating their meals with the rest of the family, they begin learning some of their first important lessons in social behavior – among them that shouting, throwing food, and trying other attention-getting tactics will be firmly dealt with.

As far as possible, they should be eating some of the same food as everyone else, even if only in puréed form. A taste of the pasta, a small serving of the vegetables, a couple of spoonfuls of stew can help make a toddler feel like one of the family. Watching other people enjoy foods will help toddlers accept them, too.

six superfoods

Millet This is the only grain that is a complete protein; it is rich in iron and other important minerals, too. Millet is also very easily digested.

Beans A great energy food that also supplies protein. Baked beans in tomato sauce with strips of whole wheat toast and a piece of fruit make great toddler meal. But choose sugar-free beans (read the label for the ingredients list).

Salmon Like other oily fish, salmon supplies quality protein as well as fats that are vital to the nerves and brain.

Yogurt Natural yogurt is rich in calcium, protein, and some important B vitamins, and it is much more easily digested than milk. The friendly bacteria supplied by yogurt also aid digestion.

Kiwis Their sharp fresh taste is quite challenging for young taste-buds. Kiwis are especially rich in vitamin C, which remains in the fruit even after lengthy storage.

Cauliflower Like all cruciferous vegetables, this will help boost resistance and protect against respiratory problems.

the eating plan

This is the age when you can teach children the good eating habits that will stay with them for the rest of their lives: the habit of drinking water or milk to quench thirst rather than fruit juice or a can of soda; the habit of eating plenty of fruit – the best possible between-meals snack (and remember that bananas are not the only fruit); and the habit of enjoying a wide range of vegetables – lightly steamed, cooked in a minimum of water, or stir-fried, and seasoned with herbs or spices to enhance their flavor.

Toddlers should be eating healthy meals now, to meet the nutritional demands of young growing bodies. They need a good breakfast to keep them going all morning, a protein-rich lunch – eggs, cottage cheese, fish, chicken, beans – and an end-of-the-day meal full of the carbohydrates that will help them sleep more soundly: rice, millet, a bowl of muesli, a baked potato.

getting round the danger foods

Sugar is top of the list of Danger Foods for this age. A toddler's palate is easily satisfied with the natural sugars in fruits and vegetables unless he learns to crave the seductive sweetness of commercial "fruit" yogurts and "fruit" drinks, breakfast cereals, cakes, cookies, and candies and chocolate.

Instead of pre-sweetened and flavored fruit yogurt, grate a little raw apple or pear, mash a banana, a peach, or a nectarine, or chop kiwis into creamy natural yogurt; try a little grated nutmeg or ground cinnamon on top. Instead of sweet cookies, offer lightly buttered oatcakes, or rye crispbread, or rice cakes. And make cakes and cookies, even the healthy, homemade kind, a treat for weekends only.

The other danger foods for children this age are soft drinks, canned or bottled. Don't have them in the house. For thirsty toddlers, the two best drinks are water and milk – choose whole, not skim, milk, and preferably organic.

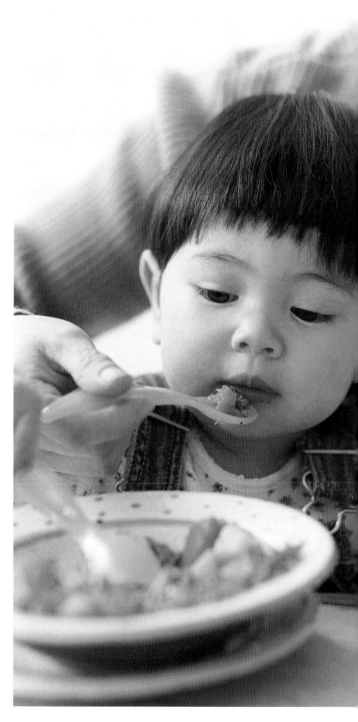

summer weekday menu plan

monday

Breakfast
Some scrambled eggs served with strips of whole wheat bread and butter. A glass of milk.

Lunch
Pasta with Avocado Sauce (see page 175). A salad of sliced tomatoes, cucumbers and shredded lettuce with a little mayonnaise. Fresh fruit.

Dinner
Chicken in a Wrap (see page 178). Yogurt with sliced peach or nectarine.

tuesday

Breakfast
Muesli with raisins and a sliced banana. Freshly squeezed orange juice.

Lunch
A salad of tuna, avocado, and tomato with a little mayonnaise and a crusty whole wheat roll and butter. A peach.

Dinner
Onion-and-Squeakburger (see page 184), spinach. Sliced kiwis.

wednesday

Breakfast
Creamy yogurt with apple purée and raisins. Whole wheat toast with butter and honey.

Lunch
Cold roast chicken with Pisto (see page 144) and a small green salad. Fresh fruit.

Dinner
Potato Cakes with Broiled Bacon (see page 171) and Green beans. A fresh peach, or nectarine.

thursday

Breakfast
Five-grain Kruska (see page 123) with yogurt and a sliced banana or some strawberries.

Lunch
Salmon Fish Cakes (see page 139) with steamed broccoli and new potatoes. A peach.

Dinner
Sugar-free baked beans on whole wheat toast. Cucumber and tomato salad. Sliced fresh pear with a little yogurt.

friday

Breakfast
Soaked dried fruit with yogurt and a little honey.

Lunch
Poached Egg and Tomato (see page 126), with new potatoes. Strips of carrot and celery. Fresh fruit.

Dinner
Minestrone with Pesto (see page 130). Oatcakes with cream cheese. An apple.

winter weekday menu plan

monday

Breakfast
Freshly squeezed orange juice. Cooked Cereal (see page 122) with milk or cream and a little honey.

Lunch
Spanish Omelette (see page 145). Celery and carrot sticks with Hummus (see page 156).

Dinner
Pumpkin Soup (see page 133) with a crusty whole wheat roll and butter. Sliced banana with yogurt.

tuesday

Breakfast
A boiled egg with strips of whole wheat toast. Freshly squeezed orange juice.

Lunch
Chickpea Veggie Burgers (see page 182). Salad of iceberg lettuce, grated apple and carrot with mayonnaise. An apple.

Dinner
Haddock Moussaka (see page 164).

wednesday

Breakfast
Lime-E-Shake (see page 124). Whole wheat toast and butter with sugar-free fruit spread.

Lunch
Spaghetti Bolognese (see page 177). Oatcakes, with sliced cheese, and a few sticks of celery.

Dinner
Irish Stew (see page 168) with steamed cauliflower. A pear.

thursday

Breakfast
Millet muesli (see page 48) with chopped banana and yogurt.

Lunch
Cauliflower and Broccoli Cheese (see page 171) and a baked potato. An apple.

Dinner
Brown Rice with Roasted Vegetables (see pages 173 and 174). Fresh fruit salad.

friday

Breakfast
Grapefruit segments. Cooked Cereal (see page 122) with milk and a little honey.

Lunch
Sugar-free baked beans on whole wheat toast. Small mixed salad. An apple.

Dinner
Leek and Watercress Soup (see page 131). A crusty whole wheat roll. Sticks of carrot and celery with Hummus (see page 156).

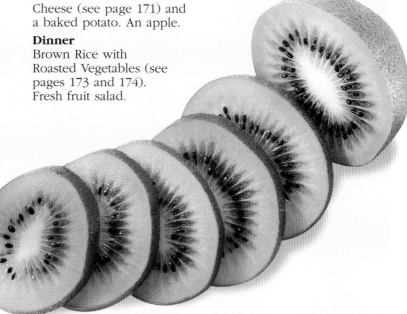

pre-school years

When they are four, children's **energy** needs **increase** dramatically. Pre-school children are physically much more active, their developing **brainpower** and mental skills are demanding, and their bodies are growing rapidly. At this age it is requisite for them to have their **calories** derived from a well-balanced intake of foods that supply adequate amounts of the essential **nutrients**.

Boys of this age will need an average of 1,700 calories a day and girls 1,550 calories, and the major nutritional trap lies in wait for the unwary parent. Because children at this age can develop voracious appetites to fuel their calorie needs, it's all too easy to submit to "pester power" and to let your children get these calories from the food sources that don't provide any benefit.

Packages of potato chips, cookies, sticky buns, sweet drinks, candy, and chocolate are an instant and easy solution. But this type of diet of high-fat, high-sugar, high-salt convenience foods carries the following three great risks:

• First, by filling children up, they displace healthy food items from the daily menu.

• Secondly, they deprive children of the life-time protection against heart disease, osteoporosis, and many forms of cancer that is provided by the "nutraceuticals" – natural chemical substances – found only in wholefoods.

• Thirdly, they encourage bad eating habits and foster addictions to salt and sugar which are likely to stay with a child for the rest of his life as well as turn him into one of today's generation of overweight children.

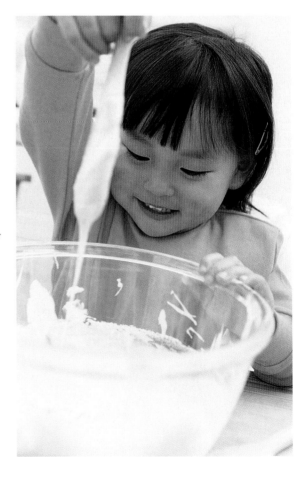

six superfoods

Bananas Whole, mashed, puréed into a milkshake, baked – however they are eaten, they provide 100 calories of supernutrition, including potassium, vitamin B_6, folic acid, and fiber.

Buckwheat Not in fact a cereal but a nut, this makes wonderful pancakes as "containers" for many other foods. Buckwheat is rich in rutin, which protects the circulatory system and helps reduce the effects of over-consumption of wheat.

Chicken Free-range and organic, of course. Quick and easy to cook and perfect protein for children. Stir-fried with vegetables or wrapped in a buckwheat pancake, it is an ultimate superfood.

Grapes Almost all children adore grapes, which are nourishing and bursting with energy.

Potatoes Another children's favorite, (but only as French fries for an occasional treat). Boiled, baked in their skins, roasted in olive oil, or mashed, they are filling and supply good levels of fiber, B vitamins, minerals, and vitamin C.

Whole wheat bread Definitely a taste to encourage as early as possible so that it becomes a child's automatic choice over the flavorless commercial white bread. Another good source of healthy calories combined with B vitamins, protein, and fiber.

the eating plan

By now your child is probably attending a playgroup or nursery school and is beginning to learn the social advantages of eating with others outside the family circle. This is a vital period for building social skills and for broadening taste and texture sensations which combine to produce the joy of eating.

As a toddler, your child has already learned to join in with the occasional family meal, and now this should be the norm rather than the special occasion. It isn't easy with busy lifestyles to have the whole family sit down together at any meal of the day, but at least try for regular family breakfasts, even if it does mean a slightly earlier start. The benefit will be worth the effort. Why

not plan as well to reinstate the Sunday family dinner, a practice which is sadly declining.

Interestingly, in areas of the country where children's diets tend to be much healthier, family meals are not confined to special occasions, like Christmas Day and Thanksgiving, but are still an essential part of the pattern of family life.

the danger foods

The danger foods for four- to five-year-olds are still the high-sugar snacks, breakfast cereals, and soft drinks that you have been keeping from your toddler. If you don't buy them they can't eat them – and they're not healthy at any age.

summer weekday menu plan

monday

Breakfast
Muesli (see page 120).

Lunch
Fishy Feast (see page 139) with whole wheat bread and butter. A small bunch of seedless grapes.

Dinner
Vegetable Couscous (see page 172). Mashed banana with yogurt and honey.

tuesday

Breakfast
Banana-to-Go breakfast in a mug (see page 124), with one slice of whole wheat toast and butter.

Lunch
Minestrone with Rice and Tomatoes (see page 130), with a whole wheat roll. Greek yogurt.

Dinner
Rosti-topped Fish Pie (see page 167), with peas. Stewed apple with a little crème fraîche.

wednesday

Breakfast
French Toast (see page 126). A small apple, sliced.

Lunch
Savory Egg (see page 153), with strips of whole wheat toast for dipping. A banana.

Dinner
Pasta Salad with Tuna (see page 147). A bunch of seedless grapes.

thursday

Breakfast
A poached egg on a slice of lightly buttered whole wheat toast. A tangerine.

Lunch
Granny Smith's Welsh Rarebit (see page 155). A small salad of chopped tomato and avocado.

Dinner
Split Pea and Rice Soup (see page 134). Upside-down Pudding (see page 188).

friday

Breakfast
Fruitfast (see page 124), served with thick Greek yogurt and a little honey. A warm whole wheat roll and butter with organic jam (additive-free).

Lunch
Baked potato filled with baked beans. Fresh berries with natural yogurt and a little honey.

Dinner
Potato Cakes with Broiled Bacon (see page 171). (Note: if your child does not like bacon or smoked ham, use unsmoked ham, or thin strips of stir-fried chicken breast instead.) Purée of fresh strawberries and mascarpone cheese.

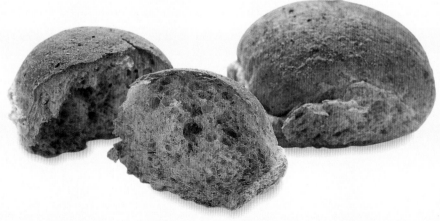

winter weekday menu plan

monday

Breakfast
Plain Pancakes (see page 190, omit sugar), served wrapped around a ripe banana.

Lunch
Marinated Broiled Chicken (see page 138), with any green vegetable.

Dinner
Macaroni mixed with cooked diced carrot and broccoli, and a tomato sauce (see page 176). Small bowl of apple purée with custard.

tuesday

Breakfast
Barley Cakes (see page 127), filled with a mixture of cottage cheese and seedless raisins.

Lunch
Spanish Omelette (see page 145), served with shredded lettuce, cucumber, and a few cherry tomatoes.

Dinner
Real Fish Strips (see page 166), with mashed potato and corn. Peeled sliced kiwis.

wednesday

Breakfast
Scrambled Egg with Tomatoes and Mushrooms (see page 125) on whole wheat toast.

Lunch
Cauliflower and Broccoli Cheese (see page 171). A ripe pear.

Dinner
Vegetable Couscous (see page 172) with a few tiny pieces of chicken fried together with the onion. A few slices of peeled fresh mango.

thursday

Breakfast
Real Fruity Yogurt (see page 123), with a hot whole wheat roll and a slice of Edam cheese.

Lunch
Pita Plus (see page 149). A tangerine and a few grapes.

Dinner
Tuna Mash (see page 152), with carrots and French beans. A Blueberry Muffin (see page 162).

friday

Breakfast
Cooked Cereal (see page 122), with one slice of whole wheat toast and butter.

Lunch
Indian Kidney Beans (see page 185).

Dinner
Poached Chicken (see page 166). Organic fruit yogurt.

off to school

Small bodies need **good nourishment** to get them through the school day. Children's brains are even hungrier than their bodies, voracious in their need for **oxygen**, **energy**, and **key nutrients**, especially **iron**, **magnesium**, and the **B vitamins**. If these demands are not met, children will find it difficult to learn, remember, and pay attention.

Hard to believe? Not for the teachers and pupils at 803 state schools in New York City. From 1979 to 1982 changes were made gradually to cafeteria menus in those schools. Out went soft drinks, sweet-vending machines, high-sugar snacks, and artificial food colors. In came fresh fruit and salad, and whole wheat rolls, pasta, and pizzas. Over the four years, the academic performance of two million pupils in those schools, assessed by the US California Achievement Test, rose from 11 percent below the national average to 5 percent above it. And the most dramatic improvements were seen in "learning-disabled" children.

If the school your child is now attending hosts soft-drink and sugary snack vending machines; if the lunchtime menu features pies, desserts, and French fries; if whole wheat bread, fresh fruit, and salads are conspicuous by their absence – take the matter in your own hands and organize a protest among like-minded parents.

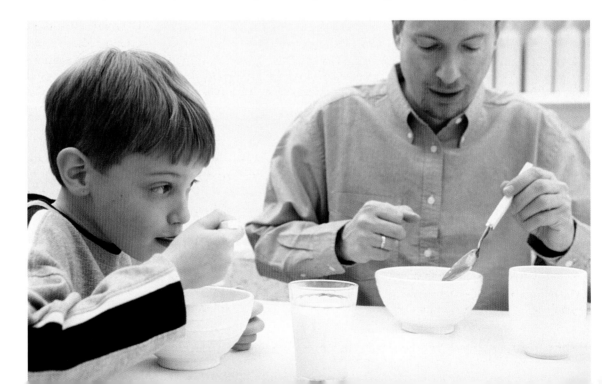

six superfoods

Apple A tasty, crunchy apple supplies energy, improves resistance, does wonders for the digestive system, and nourishes nerves. Its skin is especially nutrient-rich.

Dried fruit Dates, figs, raisins, golden raisins, are nourishing and energizing, assist digestion, and supply useful minerals like iron and calcium.

Oats Good for providing nourishment for the complete nervous system. Cooked oatmeal is an ideal breakfast food for school-children.

Eggs Supply protein, iron, zinc, and calcium, plus vitamin A to build resistance, and vitamin E. Choose free-range or organic eggs.

Sardines Another great brain-food, because they are loaded with iron and zinc plus lots of calcium. Persuade children to enjoy eating the bones.

Whole wheat bread Includes rolls, pita breads, or crackers. A school-child's diet needs the protein, vitamins, minerals, and fiber generously supplied by whole wheat.

the eating plan

If children eat a nourishing breakfast, their school day is off to a flying start. But if breakfast is a quick "fruit" drink and a couple of cookies or one of the sugar-laden "healthy" breakfast cereals, yoyo-ing blood sugar levels (see Carbohydrates, pages 12–13) will play havoc with concentration and alertness. This is because the brain needs 70 percent of the body's blood-sugar supplies. By break-time kids will be desperate for a sugar-fix.

Most schools provide a sit-down midday meal. If you or your child prefer food from home, pack an appealing lunchbox. Always include a piece of fruit, a small carton of a favorite salad with a plastic fork, small packages of nuts, if permitted, or dried fruit for snacking, perhaps a healthy (low fat) granola bar; and sandwiches, rolls, or pita pockets with some form of protein – eggs, fish, chicken – for filling.

It is a good idea to check if your child's school has guidelines about packed lunches. They may ban nuts or peanut butter, for instance, because of possible dangers to children allergic to them (see page 44).

Most children come home from school tired and hungry. They need to relax and have something to drink and a bite to eat. In the summer, consider dips with a choice of crunchy vegetables or breadsticks for dipping; or a fresh fruit salad or a fruit smoothie (yogurt blended with fresh fruit) in the summer. In winter, offer a fruit purée and a muffin or whole wheat cinnamon toast as a special treat.

a good last meal of the day

Too much supper, including food that is too rich and eaten too late, can be a recipe for sleeplessness. Get children to nibble fresh carrot or celery sticks when they sit down and include a green vegetable in the menu. In winter, think of thick vegetable soups with garlic croutons, in summer a simple salad. Fish cakes, meat, or vegetable burgers, baked potatoes with cottage cheese, or baked beans on toast are other ideas.

For drinks, choose whole organic milk – a glassful at breakfast and supper, water, or fruit juice diluted with plenty of water. Tea and coffee are inappropriate for children of this age.

The danger foods for this age group are potato chips and soft drinks, which your children may be encountering through school for the first time. Don't get critical if they ask for these new treats – just make it plain that "treats" are exactly what they are, and only to be enjoyed on special occasions.

summer weekday menu plan

monday

Breakfast
Whole wheat cereal with milk. A banana.

Lunch
Minestrone with Rice and Tomatoes (see page 130). Cucumber and cottage-cheese salad. A peach or nectarine.

Dinner
Dips with crunchy vegetables (see page 149). Riceburger (see page 183) with French beans. Pieces of fresh fruit.

tuesday

Breakfast
Fruitfast (see page 124) with muesli.

Lunch
Tuna Eggs Mayonnaise (see page 196). Green salad with tomatoes and cucumber.

Dinner
Sardines on toast. Pancakes (see page 190) rolled with a little sugar-free fruit spread.

wednesday

Breakfast
Poached Egg and Tomato (see page 126).

Lunch
Pizza Baguette (see page 154), with cucumber and lettuce salad. A peach or nectarine.

Dinner
Sophie's Indonesian Vegetable Stew (see page 178). Yogurt with fresh fruit mixed into it.

thursday

Breakfast
Freshly squeezed orange juice. Boiled egg with a slice of whole wheat toast and butter.

Lunch
Real Fish Sticks (see page 166) with boiled new potatoes. A salad of grated raw carrot, beets, and slices of tomato with a little mayonnaise.

Dinner
Brown Rice (see page 173) with cheese. Salad of watercress and chicory. Fresh fruit.

friday

Breakfast
Muesli with raisins, soaked overnight in apple juice, served with yogurt.

Lunch
Spanish Omelette (see page 145) with French beans. A peach or nectarine.

Dinner
Pasta with Tomato and Red Pepper Sauce (see page 176). Salad of lettuce and cucumber. Greek yogurt with strawberries.

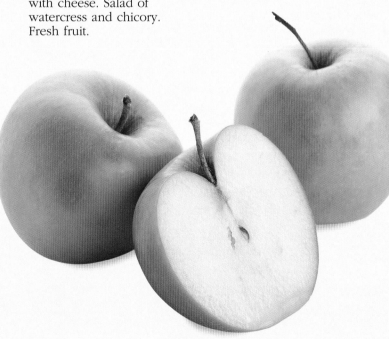

winter weekday menu plan

monday

Breakfast
Cooked Cereal (see page 122) with honey and a little cream.

Lunch
Bean Burger (see page 184) with Coleslaw (see page 198). An apple.

Dinner
Real Fish Sticks (see page 166), Mashed Potatoes and Celeriac (see page 180) and peas. Stewed pears with yogurt.

tuesday

Breakfast
Scrambled Egg with Tomatoes and Mushrooms (see page 125) and whole wheat toast.

Lunch
Quick Spinach Snack (see page 154). Oatcakes with butter and sticks of celery. An apple.

Dinner
Baked potato with baked beans. Soaked prunes and apricots with yogurt.

wednesday

Breakfast
Cooked Cereal (see page 122) with milk or cream. Whole wheat toast with butter and sugar-free fruit spread.

Lunch
South of France Omelette (page 169). Whole wheat roll and butter. A pear.

Dinner
Baked Savoy Cabbage Soup (see page 132). Sticks of celery and carrot with Hummus (see page 156). Stewed apple with yogurt.

thursday

Breakfast
Boiled egg with whole wheat toast and butter.

Lunch
Veggie Burger with Spinach Cheese Topping (see page 182). Coleslaw (see page 198).

Dinner
Roast chicken with Mashed Potatoes and Celeriac (see page 180). A baked apple stuffed with dried fruit.

friday

Breakfast
A tangerine. Whole wheat cereal, such as Five-grain Kruska (see page 123), with a dollop of yogurt and a sliced banana.

Lunch
Salmon Fish Cakes (see page 139), with puréed spinach. An apple.

Dinner
Broccoli and Anchovy Pasta (see page 175). Rice cakes with cream cheese and celery sticks.

Lunchbox ideas

On school days, if your child wishes to take a lunch to school. These ideas for packed lunches ensure healthy food in the middle of the day.

• Hummus (see page 156), alfalfa sprouts, and tomato sandwiches on whole wheat bread. A small package of raisins. A piece of fresh fruit.

• Tuna and cucumber sandwiches with mayonnaise on whole wheat bread. A bunch of seedless grapes. A low fat granola bar.

• Cold chicken and lettuce with mayonnaise in a whole wheat roll. A package of dried fruit. A banana.

• Sardines mashed with a little mayonnaise and one or two lettuce leaves in whole wheat bread. A small container of Coleslaw (see page 198) – don't forget the fork! An apple.

• Tuna salad with corn, tomato, and chopped parsley in a little container. A low-fat granola bar. A piece of fresh fruit.

the years of growth

The period from nine to 13 is an indeterminate, **in-between time** for children: they are in between being children but not quite yet young adults, just beginning their passage through puberty. Although **nutrition** is vital at every age, there are special needs during this period of **growth** and **development into maturity.**

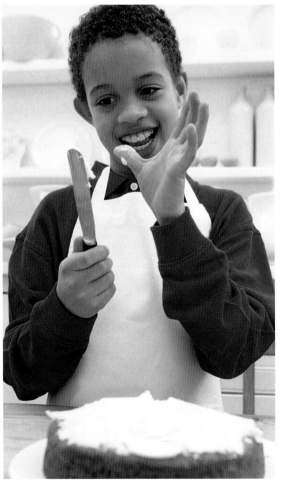

By now your children will be insisting on making many of their own food choices, and the decisions they make can be crucial. What they eat now has a profound effect on their day-to-day quality of life and performance, but it is also a key determining factor of their long-term health.

Good nutrition at this stage is a two-pronged attack on many of the illnesses which are often regarded as the inevitable consequences of aging. First, good nutrition ensures an abundant intake of the protective nutrients that guard against heart and circulatory disease, premature senility, and osteoporosis. Second, nutritious eating avoids high consumption of damaging foods like saturated animal fats, trans-fats, salt, sugar, and all the products of the commercial junk-food industry.

You won't achieve this balanced way of eating by heavy-handedness or prohibition. The way to instill good eating habits that will last your children a lifetime is by setting a good example yourself, encouraging an interest in food, and getting children into the kitchen. Take time to teach them the simple basics of cooking, and make sure they do their bit by involving them in food preparation, setting the table, and doing the dishes.

Most children of this age enjoy the creative process of cooking, and as long as you teach them properly, they are perfectly safe in the kitchen with appropriate supervision.

six superfoods

Dates A healthy sweet and delicious treat which supplies plenty of much-needed iron and a good boost of potassium.

Oranges A fresh orange before any meal ups absorption of iron, calcium, and other minerals from foods, thanks to its high vitamin C content.

Cooked cereal No better start to the day, because of its iron, zinc, calcium, and B vitamins.

Lentils A great source of protein which also supply iron and zinc.

Fish An excellent source of protein, but include oily as well as white fish to guarantee sufficient intake of essential fatty acids.

Eggs Free-range or organic – the most natural convenience food of all. Cheap, quick, easy, and full of protein and B vitamins.

the eating plan

During this period of rapid growth and development, both boys and girls need a massive input of energy. Ideally, aim for six daily servings of starchy foods like rice, whole wheat bread, potatoes, pasta, and whole wheat cereals; five portions of fruit and vegetables; and two portions each of dairy products and non-dairy proteins, animal or vegetable. The wider the variety of food selections, the broader the spectrum of vitamins, minerals, trace elements, and the other highly protective phytonutrients that your children will consume. It cannot be reiterated often enough that this is the vital time to establish healthy eating habits that will stay with your children for life.

Try to keep your children's comsumption of fried and high-sugar foods to a minimum so they become occasional treats rather than their staple diet. The high-calorie, low-nutrient value of many convenience foods pushes aside the consumption of healthier nutrients. Studies in America show that some youngsters in this age group are getting in excess of 45 percent of their calories from fat, making them prime candidates for heart disease and strokes in later life.

You must, however, beware of fanaticism which could turn children into total rebels who stuff themselves with junk at every opportunity when you're not watching, or you of risking malnutrition in your children by being obsessive about organic foods and whole wheat cereals. There are already parents so phobic about agricultural chemicals that they would rather their children went without fresh produce if organic isn't available.

danger foods for pre-teens
Salt, caffeine, and canned soft drinks can all interfere with a child's absorption of calcium from the diet. High bran foods have the same effect and can also reduce the absorption of iron. For girls of this age, particularly, building up stores of iron is vital before their periods start.

summer weekday menu plan

monday

Breakfast
Sardines on Toast: mash sardines with a little vinegar, spread on a slice of whole wheat toast, cover with thin slices of tomato and heat under the broiler. Serve with a spoonful of ketchup. Serve a second slice of whole wheat toast with butter and honey.

Lunch
Hot Pancetta Savories (see page 154), served with a mixed salad.

Dinner
Zoë's Shrimp and Vegetable Stir-fry (see page 164). Summer Pudding (see page 188).

tuesday

Breakfast
Muesli (see page 120). Chunk of warm whole wheat French bread, with a small piece of mild cheese.

Lunch
Fish Soup (see page 135). This may seem a lot of trouble for lunch, but simply reheat from a previous batch and omit the rouille and croûtons. Serve with crusty whole wheat rolls. Follow with sliced oranges sprinkled with chopped dates and natural yogurt.

Dinner
Homemade chicken burger: combine ground chicken with finely chopped onion and raw egg; shape into thin burgers and cook under a hot broiler until cooked right through. Serve on a bed of lettuce with tomatoes, ketchup, relish, and oven French fries. Creamy Fruit Tart (see page 186).

wednesday

Breakfast
Lime-E-Shake (see page 124), served with 2 slices whole wheat toast, butter and honey.

Lunch
Smoked Mackerel Quiche (see page 140), served with a tomato, watercress, and cucumber salad.

Dinner
Minestrone (see page 128), served with bread, cheese, and an apple.

thursday

Breakfast
Salmon Fishcakes (see page 139). These are great served cold for breakfast within a day or two of making. Serve with thin slices of whole wheat bread and butter.

Lunch
Colcannon (see page 141). Sliced melon and sliced fresh orange.

Dinner
Chicken Salad with Honey and Chili (see page 138). Any fresh fruit.

friday

Breakfast
2 boiled eggs, served with 2 slices whole wheat toast and butter. Half a grapefruit.

Lunch
Bread and Tomato Salad (see page 147). 1 kiwifruit, peeled and chopped into a carton of natural yogurt.

Dinner
Broccoli and Anchovy Pasta (see page 175). Fruit Dipped in Chocolate Sauce (see page 186).

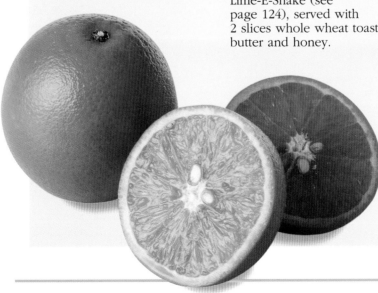

winter weekday menu plan

monday

Breakfast
Cooked Cereal (see page 122), with 2 slices whole wheat toast and butter. A banana.

Lunch
Spinach Soufflé (see page 152). Selection of presoaked dried fruits.

Dinner
Herbed Kofta Kebabs (see page 169), with rice and peas. Upside-down Pudding (see page 188).

tuesday

Breakfast
Poached Egg and Tomato (see page 126) and crispy broiled bacon with a slice of whole wheat toast.

Lunch
Fish Cakes (see page 153), served with a large beefsteak tomato sliced thinly and drizzled with a little olive oil.

Dinner
Pumpkin Soup (see page 133). Granny Smith's Welsh Rarebit (see page 155).

wednesday

Breakfast
Oatmeal Bannocks (see page 127); serve some with jam, some with cheese.

Lunch
Vegetable Curry with Dal (see page 181), served with a chapatti or pita bread.

Dinner
Marinated Broiled Chicken (see page 138), served with any broiled or steamed vegetables. Real Rice Pudding (see page 191).

thursday

Breakfast
Old-fashioned Kedgeree (see page 140): a substantial breakfast dish, ideal if this is a busy day for school sports.

Lunch
Pizza Baguette (see page 154). A ripe pear.

Dinner
Irish Stew (see page 168), served with a mixture of puréed rutabaga and parsnip. Fresh fruit.

friday

Breakfast
Baked beans on a helping of Bubble and Squeak (see page 174). Half a grapefruit or a fresh orange.

Lunch
Spanish Omelette (see page 145), served with a small green salad.

Dinner
Any fresh fish fillet, broiled with tomatoes and served with boiled potatoes and any green vegetable. Blackberry and Apple Crumble (see page 189).

Lunchbox ideas
At this age, lunches at home are mainly for weekends or school holidays. Preparing lunchboxes for school becomes very important. The suggestions here provide nutritious food that's great to eat.

- Hard-boiled egg. A tomato. A whole wheat buttered roll. A few dates. A carton of Greek yogurt.

- Pita bread filled with a mixture of tuna, chopped apple, a little natural yogurt, and a teaspoon of lemon juice. A thick slice of Green Tea Bread (see page 161).

- A small carton of fresh orange juice. A sandwich of thinly sliced chicken breast and thinly sliced red pepper, spread with mayonnaise and sprinkled with torn basil leaves, on whole wheat bread. Apricot Scone (see page 159).

- Selection of Stuffed Celery Sticks (see page 155). A tangerine. A package of vegetable fries. A carton of natural yogurt.

- Two thin slices of Banana and Walnut Bread (see page 163), made into a sandwich with a slice of Edam cheese. A ripe pear, a package of nuts and raisins, and a small bar of organic chocolate.

the turbulent teens

For today's children, the teen years can be both exciting and stressful. Settling down happily in a wider world, much of it centered at a large school, with its crowd of new classmates, term papers, and exams, requires the sort of self-confidence and energy that can be greatly boosted by good nutrition at home.

Both inside and outside of school, there's a very competitive world, where looks and possessions can take on huge importance, and of course, there's the stress of puberty with its hormonal upheavals.

For all these reasons, children need the very best nourishment to help them deal with these challenges and to meet the huge demands of growth and puberty. Sadly, it is for this age group particularly that junk food with all its anti-nutrients tends to become part of everyday life, and hamburgers, French fries, and a soft drink from a can constitute normal social eating. It is at this age that sound eating habits learned around the family table will really prove their value.

six superfoods

Oats Packed with enough B vitamins to make them first-class, nourishing nerves and preventing exhaustion, oats are just the food for teenagers. They're also high in zinc (vital for active minds and clear skins), iron for stamina, calcium for healthy bones, and magnesium for tranquillity.

Canned salmon An excellent source of the vital fats needed for brains, nerves, and skin especially. Rich in bone-building calcium.

Watercress Slip a little watercress into salads, soups, and sandwiches: it is rich in protective factors as well as useful minerals.

Sesame and sunflower seeds
Like nuts, these are excellent sources of protein. Eat them at the same time as vitamin C-rich foods for good absorption. These two seeds in particular are high in zinc, vital for puberty (see Eating Disorders, page 213).

Chicken Cold roast chicken is good grazing food for hungry teenagers who don't want to sit down for meals; low in fat, it supplies good protein, zinc, and B vitamins.

Apples Keep a bowl of apples on the kitchen table for a super-healthy between-meals snack.

the eating plan

Much of the time, as the teenage years go by, your children will be eating and drinking away from home – lunching in the school cafeteria, socializing, going out on the town. It is your job to make sure that the meals they *do* eat at home make up for any deficiencies there may be in what they are eating elsewhere.

Breakfast, hopefully, will by now be established as a meal which the family eats together. Make cooked cereal in winter; in summer, serve wonderful muesli with sunflower and sesame seeds, soaked overnight, to which you add a little cream and a few berries. Try, too, to make a point of having at least one evening a week that is designated a family meal together. And as far as possible, weekend midday meals should be more occasions for relaxed eating at home.

healthy snacking

Many parents cannot be bothered to put up with constant invasion by strange teenagers dropping by for meals or snacks at all hours. But if your home is an open house for your children's friends, not only will you see much more of them, you'll also have the pleasure of meeting those friends. And you'll have the chance to see that on these occasions, too, your children are eating food that is healthy as well as delicious.

Grazing seems to be an established habit of modern teenagers. If your refrigerator and pantry are junk-food-free, healthy snacking is what they'll be doing. See pages 182–84 for recipes for several burgers they could find in the freezer any time,

along with whole wheat rolls. Tomato or meat sauce from the freezer are the makings of a quick pasta; they should also be able to find at any time in cabinets or the refrigerator, plenty of fresh fruit, carrot and celery sticks, cottage cheese, hard cheese, hummus, eggs, canned sardines and tuna, and natural yogurt.

the danger foods

Limitless potato chips and soft drinks – the latter usually with artificial sweeteners, since many teenagers are on semi-permanent diets – are the danger foods most likely to prove irresistible to teenagers, because they are probably what the rest of the gang will be enjoying. Your children should know by now that these are treats that will have to come out of their own pocket money. They should also know that artificial sweeteners may be a serious health risk. In fact, by this time they should be savvy enough to read the small print on lists of ingredients without any urging from you.

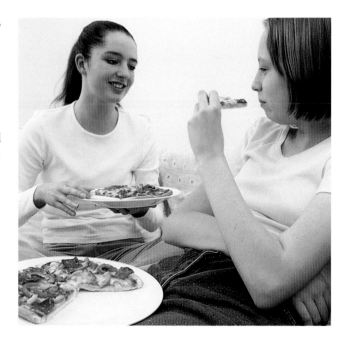

summer weekday menu plan

monday

Breakfast
Muesli with sunflower and sesame seeds, soaked overnight in water, served with yogurt and a few raspberries or strawberries.

Lunch
Savory Eggs (see page 153). Whole wheat roll and butter. Fresh fruit.

Dinner
Cold roast chicken with new potatoes. Tomato and cucumber salad. Fresh fruit.

tuesday

Breakfast
Banana-to-Go (see page 124).

Lunch
Bean Burgers (see page 184) with a green salad. Fresh fruit.

Dinner
Zoë's Shrimp and Vegetable Stir-fry (see page 164). Stewed pears and yogurt.

wednesday

Breakfast
Scrambled Egg with Tomatoes and Mushrooms (see page 125). Whole wheat toast with butter.

Lunch
Minestrone (see page 128) with a crusty whole wheat roll. Salad of avocado, tomato, and cottage cheese with chopped chives or cilantro.

Dinner
Pasta with Avocado Sauce (see page 175). Spinach purée. Fresh fruit.

thursday

Breakfast
Five-grain Kruska (see page 123).

Lunch
Spanish Omelette (see page 145). Green salad. Fresh fruit.

Dinner
Black Bean Chili (see page 168), with green beans. Rice cakes with cheese. A pear.

friday

Breakfast
Boiled egg with whole wheat toast. A peach.

Lunch
Real Fish Sticks (see page 166) with some new potatoes and a green salad. Fresh fruit.

Dinner
Veggie Burgers with Spinach Cheese Topping (see page 182). Braised fennel. Summer fruits with yogurt.

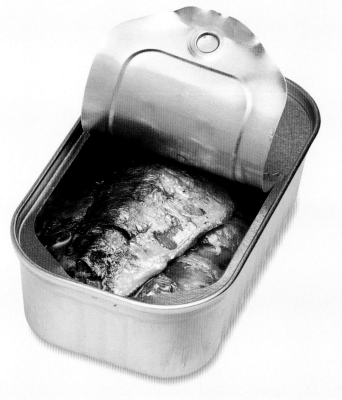

winter weekday menu plan

monday

Breakfast
Oatmeal Bannocks (see page 127); accompanied by apple purée.

Lunch
Brown Rice (see page 173) with chopped summer vegetables. Chicory and watercress salad.

Dinner
Grilled chicken with mashed potato and braised leeks. Soaked dried fruit with yogurt.

tuesday

Breakfast
Fruitfast (see page 124) with Greek yogurt.

Lunch
Sardines on toast. Coleslaw (see page 198).

Dinner
Celery, carrot, and fennel sticks with Hummus (see page 156). Rabbit with Prunes (see page 166), served with a baked potato and spinach purée. A dessert (pages 186–91).

wednesday

Breakfast
Cooked Cereal (see page 122) cooked with raisins, served with milk or cream.

Lunch
Hot Pancetta Savories (see page 154). Sticks of carrot and celery with cream cheese. An apple.

Dinner
Salmon Fish Cakes (see page 139) with carrots and green beans. Baked apple stuffed with ground almonds.

thursday

Breakfast
Freshly pressed orange juice. Baked Eggs and Bacon (see page 125). Whole wheat toast.

Lunch
Granny Smith's Welsh Rarebit (see page 155). Chicory and watercress salad. A pear.

Dinner
Pasta with Classic Bolognese Sauce (see page 177). Stir-fried cauliflower and broccoli.

friday

Breakfast
Whole wheat cereal with a sliced banana and yogurt.

Lunch
Savory Eggs (see page 153). A green salad, whole wheat roll, and slices of cheese.

Dinner
Beanburger (see page 184) with Broccoli with Spinach (see page 180). Pancakes (see page 190) filled with apple purée.

Lunchbox ideas

There are many times – school trips and sports events, for instance – when teens need a good packed lunch. Here are some nutrient-filled suggestions.

• Peanut butter and banana sandwiches on whole wheat bread. A banana. A low fat granola bar.

• A carton of tuna, tomato, and mayonnaise salad. A whole wheat roll with lettuce, and cucumber. An apple.

• A whole wheat roll filled with cold chicken, tomato, and lettuce, with mayonnaise. A small bar of dark organic chocolate. A package of nuts and raisins.

• Watercress, carrot, and cucumber sandwiches with mayonnaise on whole wheat bread. Cheese Pretzels (see page 157). An apple.

• A whole wheat roll filled with chicory and a sardine-and-mayonnaise mixture. A banana. A slice of Carrot Cake (see page 163).

vegetarian children

Unless parents are vegetarian themselves, a child's decision to **become a vegetarian** frequently causes panic and brings dire words of warning from the family doctor. In fact, being a **good vegetarian** can be much healthier than being a meat-eater – **less** heart disease, **fewer** strokes, **less** high blood pressure, **less** bowel cancer, and **less** obesity.

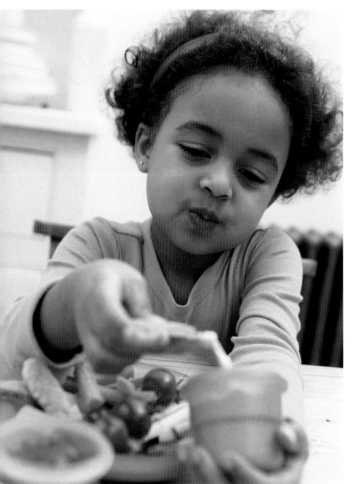

While a simple vitamin and mineral supplement is often a good idea for children, many nutritionists think that it is essential for vegetarians. Buying the appropriate product for their age will make sure that children on a completely meat-free diet do not become deficient in vitamin B_{12} and iron.

Unfortunately, if your child simply gives up eating meat, fish, and chicken and lives on little else except bread, cheese, eggs, and junk food, you've got a recipe for disaster. Such children need to be persuaded to take a greater interest in eating more nutritious and healthy foods. One of the best ways of encouraging healthier eating for vegetarian children, and, in fact, of persuading virtually any child to eat some fresh produce, is by getting them to grow their own.

Naturally, a garden is great and if you've got one give an area of it to your children. Even without a garden spot, however, your kids can grow their own produce in pots on a terrace or balcony or even in a window box. And once they have planted the seed, nurtured their crop, and harvested the result they'll want to eat it.

six superfoods

Radishes These are favorites of children because they grow so quickly. Sow small amounts regularly in a window box. Radishes are a great aid to digestion, and they protect the liver.

Carrots These are easy if you've got good soil in the garden; otherwise plant them in tubs or window boxes. Bursting with beta-carotene for skin, eyesight, and strong natural resistance.

Green beans Use one of the dwarf bush varieties. These will grow well in a large window box but would probably be better in a large pot or half-barrel.

Cherry tomatoes Another all-time children's favorite. The bush variety will grow abundantly in a hanging basket. Rich in vitamin C and the unique cancer- and heart disease-protective nutrient lycopene.

Lettuce Your children will never turn their noses up at lettuce again once they've grown some for themselves. Grow the mixed "cut and come again" varieties in a window box. The darker the color lettuce you grow, the richer it is in nutrients.

Zucchini Give a vegetarian child (or any other child) a bush zucchini variety to plant in a half-barrel and he'll be itching to take the first ripe one to school to show it off to friends.

Vegetarian children need to get their protein from varied sources. While eggs and cheese are quick and easy, it is essential that you also feed them a mixture of cereals and legumes. Soybeans and their by-products like tofu, soy cheese, and soy granules are an excellent protein source with the added benefits of the plant hormones that protect against cancer, heart disease, and osteoporosis.

the eating plan

It's very important to be organized with a vegetarian diet, and for this reason you should pay particular attention to what you have in your pantry. Make sure you always keep on hand plenty of canned beans, lots of dried pasta, rice, lentils, chickpeas, nuts, seeds, and dried fruits. With these available you can always rustle up a protein-rich meal, even if you haven't had time to get to the supermarket.

School meals can be a particular problem for vegetarians, since children often end up with only a plate of French fries and, if you're lucky, a small, uninteresting salad. The increasing availability of ethnic foods in schools has, however, made things easier, since dishes like vegetable curries, dal, vegetarian lasagnas, pizzas, and even veggieburgers are more often available.

In winter, thick soups and root vegetable casseroles with beans and rice guarantee warming calories and body-building nutrients without relying on high fat cakes, rich desserts, and other unhealthy foods.

the danger foods

The major risk for vegetarian children is that they fill up their calorie needs with large amounts of cakes, cookies, and potato chips. These all have poor nutritional value in relation to their high calorie content and easily lead to excessive weight gain. The other great danger is that in some young girls turning vegetarian may become a cover for eating disorders. It's all too easy to refuse food on the grounds of vegetarianism when the real reason could be anorexia nervosa (see pages 211–12).

summer weekday menu plan

monday

Breakfast
Muesli (see page 120).
A whole wheat roll with
butter and either jam or
honey.

Lunch
Roasted Vegetables (see
page 174) with Brown Rice
(see page 173). A fresh
sliced peach.

Dinner
Sophie's Indonesian
Vegetable Stew (see
page 178), served with
basmati rice and a mixed
salad. A favorite ice cream
and fresh pineapple.

tuesday

Breakfast
Creamy Yogurt with Nuts
and Honey (see page 123)
(no nuts for the under
fives). A slice of melon
and a croissant.

Lunch
Mashed Potato and
Celeriac (see page 180).
Fresh celery with cottage
cheese.

Dinner
Shepherdless pie: use
TVP granules instead of
ground beef and serve
with zucchini, cauliflower,
and baby fava beans.
Fresh fruit and a small
piece of cheese.

wednesday

Breakfast
Mushrooms and tomatoes
on toast: put a handful of
button mushrooms in a
small saucepan with a tiny
piece of butter and heat
gently. As soon as liquid
starts coming out of the
mushrooms, cover and
cook for 5 minutes. Add
a small can of chopped
tomatoes, stir until warm,
and serve on a thick slice
of whole wheat toast.

Lunch
Cauliflower and Broccoli
Cheese (see page 171).
Serving of any fresh berries
with a tablespoon of
cottage cheese.

Dinner
Veggieburger (see page
182) in a sesame bun with
lettuce, tomato, ketchup,
and green relish. Serve
with oven-baked sweet-
potato fries: cut sweet
potato into large strips,
brush with olive oil and
bake in a hot oven for
about 30 minutes, or
until cooked. Stewed
summer fruits with
custard.

thursday

Breakfast
Half a grapefruit. French
Toast (see page 126).

Lunch
Pisto (see page 144).

Dinner
Peppers Stuffed with
Quinoa (see page 144): use
organic peppers, if possible.
Tofu yogurt with fresh fruit.

friday

Breakfast
Multi-grain Pancakes (see
page 126). Bowl of fresh
fruit salad with yogurt.

Lunch
A selection of different
cheeses with whole wheat
bread. A ripe nectarine
and a few black grapes.

Dinner
Minestrone with Pesto
(see page 130). Summer
Pudding (see page 188).

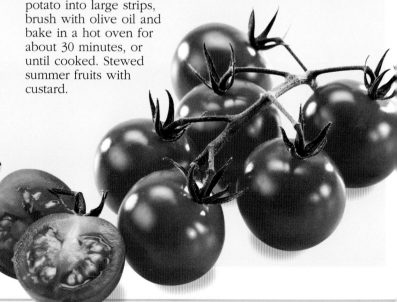

winter weekday menu plan

monday

Breakfast
Cooked Cereal (see page 122), with one of the listed additions. A wedge of warm whole wheat bread with piece of mild cheese.

Lunch
South of France Omelette (see page 169).

Dinner
High-protein Tofu Broth (see page 131). Blackberry and Apple Crumble (see page 189).

tuesday

Breakfast
Meat-free sausage brushed with olive oil and broiled with a large halved tomato.

Lunch
Black Bean Chili (see page 168). Grapes.

Dinner
Pasta with a mushroom and tomato sauce. Large mixed salad. Baked banana with honey.

wednesday

Breakfast
Scrambled Egg with Tomatoes and Mushrooms (see page 125) on whole wheat toast.

Lunch
Vegetable Samosas (see page 172), served with yogurt and mint, or tomato relish, and a small winter salad of celery, shredded lettuce and watercress.

Dinner
Broccoli with Spinach (see page 180), served with dal (see Vegetable Curry with Dal, page 181). Upside-down Pudding (see page 188).

thursday

Breakfast
Wholegrain breakfast cereal with hot milk. 2 slices of whole wheat buttered toast. A banana.

Lunch
Creamy Celery Soup (see page 131), served with thick chunks of rough country bread.

Dinner
Red Cabbage with Apple and Chestnuts (see page 181): omit the bacon and substitute vegetarian chicken or turkey slices). Baked apple stuffed with raisins, chopped dates, and honey.

friday

Breakfast
Cheese on toast: grate cheese, add a little milk, a dash of Worcester sauce and beat to a smooth cream; toast bread on one side, spread the cheese mixture on the other side and place under a hot broiler until bubbly. Serve with slices of apple.

Lunch
Broccoli with potatoes. A mixture of cashews, hazelnuts, walnuts, dried apricots, and raisins.

Dinner
Roasted Vegetables (see page 174), topped with some grated cheese and browned under the broiler for 2 minutes before serving. Ginger Fruit Pudding (see page 189).

Lunchbox ideas
• Scoop out the middle of a chunk of French bread and fill with Roasted Vegetables (see page 174). A banana, nuts, and raisins.

• A whole wheat roll spread with peanut butter, a mashed banana, and a drizzle of honey. A couple of Shortbread Trees (see page 162). An apple.

• Selection of dips (see page 149) and a bag of mixed crudités, such as carrots, celery, peppers, and cauliflower. A Blueberry Muffin (see page 162).

• A thermos of Creamy Celery Soup (see page 131) with a few chunks of ciabatta bread. A thick slice of buttered Green Tea Bread (see page 161).

• A container of Pasta Salad with Tuna (see page 147). A few Cheese Pretzels (see page 157). A small package of dried apricots, and raisins. A bunch of seedless grapes.

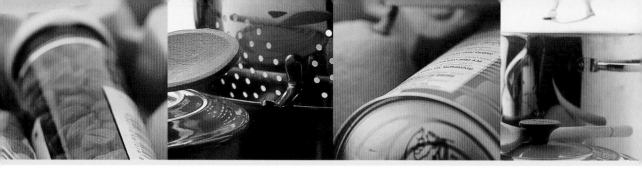

family kitchen

Your kitchen is the natural focus of family life and the place where children learn vital lessons about food choices and about eating well. Organize the kitchen and stock the cabinets carefully so that a good meal or healthy snack can always be put together, however short the notice or large the number of hungry young people.

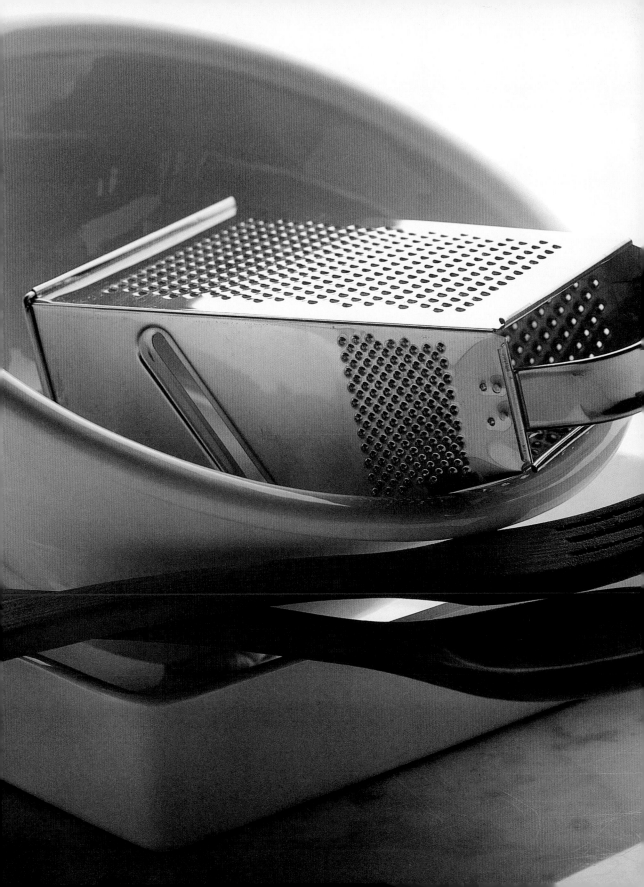

what you need

With the right pans, tools, and gadgets on your kitchen shelves and a well-planned choice of foods stored in your refrigerator, freezer, and pantry, you'll be able easily to feed the family healthily and enjoyably at any time.

pans, tools, & utensils

Saucepans
Buy the best you can afford – stainless steel will last a lifetime and is worth the investment. Saute vegetables for starting off soups and stews in the same pan you use to cook the dish, instead of using a separate pan – a useful time-saver. Avoid aluminum pans, which can be a health hazard. If you can't replace yours, do not use them to cook acidic foods such as fruit.

Non-stick saucepan
Essential for making sauces, scrambling eggs, or heating milk.

Non-stick frying pans
If possible have two: a smaller one is good for making omelettes. Make sure you use non-stick utensils with them.

Wok
This is indispensable for stir-fry dishes, which are quick, delicious, and very healthy. Classic Chinese steel woks are inexpensive, but you must follow the instructions for seasoning them. Or you may prefer a non-stick wok.

Stovetop-to-oven casseroles
These are useful for dishes that have to be started off on the top of the stove and then be transferred to the oven.

Indispensables for the kitchen drawer

Vegetable peeler

Potato masher

Kitchen scissors
Must be tough to cut up pieces of chicken.

Small whisk

Garlic crusher

Knife sharpener

Good can opener

Pasta server
A scoop with toothed sides for serving pasta, this also conveys boiled eggs from pan to plate without a spill.

Ovenproof dishes

Ovenproof earthenware dishes are useful for preparing gratins, vegetables, and bakes.

Colanders

One of your colanders should be heatproof (steel or enamel), so it can double as a steamer with a saucepan lid on top.

Salad spinner

This allows even the busiest cook to have a perfectly dry, fresh green salad every day.

Sharp kitchen knives

It's useful to have three or four, including at least one with a serrated blade for slicing soft foods such as tomatoes.

Wooden chopping boards

In various sizes. Once a week, pour boiling water over them and scrub them well.

Spatulas, pancake turners, and slotted spoons

Have a metal set and a nylon set for use with non-stick pans.

Strainers

Wooden spoons

Have several, in different sizes. Don't put wooden spoons in the dishwasher if they are favorites.

Bowls

Various, in china or Pyrex, for mixing and storage.

Lidded glass or heavy plastic containers

For storing all kinds of food in the refrigerator, so you can see them.

Measuring cups

Keep a small Pyrex measuring cup for making sauces as well as a bigger plastic one.

Set of kitchen scales

Pepper mill

One of those items that it is worth spending a little more on. Test them and choose one that does a good grinding job.

Grater

The square kind with different-sized graters on each side is the most useful. Italian cylindrical cheese graters are quick to use.

Good gadgets

Food processor

Worth its weight in gold to the harassed cook. It's indispensable for grinding meat, making breadcrumbs, chopping and grating vegetables, puréeing, mixing batters, and many other processes.

Hand-held electric mixer

Much cheaper than a food processor and almost as useful.

Electric tea kettle

Make sure it has an automatic switch-off mechanism.

Electric toaster

Juice extractor

With a good juicer you can prepare in minutes a delicious mega-dose of fresh natural goodness – especially of the vital antioxidant vitamins (see Delicious Drinks, pages 192–195).

Food mill

Try the French Mouli-legume mill; it allows you to blend and sieve at the same time, producing soups with a much more interesting texture than made by a blender or a food processor.

Herb mincer

This comprises a shallow, wooden bowl with a handled, half-moon blade – an excellent device for chopping herbs swiftly and thoroughly, without crushing them to a purée.

the pantry

Canned foods

Italian plum tomatoes: *whole tomatoes are best, rather than chopped or puréed ones.*
Chickpeas.
Sugar-free baked beans.
A variety of canned beans including soy, borlotti, kidney, and cannellini.
Tuna, sardines.

Oils

Extra-virgin olive oil and plain olive oil.
Lighter oils, such as sunflower oil or peanut oil (see page 44).
Sesame oil: *for wok cooking.*

Sauces and condiments

Shoyu, or a naturally fermented soy sauce.
Worcestershire sauce.
White-wine vinegar or cider vinegar.
Salt: *sea salt is incomparably superior in flavor to ordinary table salt.*
Low-salt stock cubes or vegetable bouillon powder.
Tomato purée in a tube.
Low- or no-sugar anchovy paste.

Organic jellies, jams, and preserves without additives, and sugar-free fruit spreads: *once opened, keep in the refrigerator.*
Good-quality pesto: *once opened, keep in the refrigerator.*

Grains and pasta

Wholewheat and unbleached white flour, all-purpose flour and self-rising.
Rice – brown, short-grain, long-grain and basmati.
Bulgur wheat.
Pasta – normal and some whole wheat: *make sure it is made from 100 percent durum wheat, as other varieties can become gummy while cooking.*
Steel-cut oats.

Herbs

Fresh herbs give a terrific boost to your cooking. Keep small pots of fresh herbs on the kitchen windowsill. Parsley: *best fresh, but it freezes well.* Mint, chives, and basil: *should always be used fresh.* Rosemary, sage, oregano, thyme, and bay leaves: *ideally should be used fresh, but are satisfactory dried.*

Dried herbs and spices can deteriorate quickly in storage. They are best kept in the dark, and should be regularly checked for use-by dates and replaced if necessary. Stale herbs and spices do nothing for your cooking.

Spices

Chili powder or crushed, dried chilies.
Paprika.
Whole nutmeg.
Black peppercorns: *freshly ground is best; pre-ground pepper is a useful stand-by but the flavor is not as good.*
Whole cinnamon sticks and ground cinnamon.
Coriander and cumin, both ground: *renew them when they lose their aromas.*
Whole cloves.
Ground ginger and preserved ginger pieces in syrup: *one teaspoon or so of the syrup can spice up sauces and desserts.*
Turmeric.
Curry powder, mild, medium, or hot, according to your preference: *don't keep it too long, since it loses its flavor rapidly.*

the vegetable rack and fruit bowl

Vegetables

Potatoes and onions: *store these in brown-paper, not plastic, bags away from light and heat. Be sure to use them before they begin to sprout.*

Garlic: *store in a porous earthenware container to keep it in good condition.*
Avocados: *store in brown-paper bags for quick ripening if they're still hard when you buy them.*

Fruit

Apples, pears.
Bananas.
Kiwis.
Oranges, grapefruit.
Lemons.

the refrigerator

Cheese

Piece of good-quality Cheddar or other hard, mild cheese.
Fresh Parmesan cheese, either a chunk or ready-grated: *buy this from a reliable delicatessen.*
Fromage frais and cottage cheese.

Salads and vegetables

Iceberg lettuce: *keeps well, so is a good salad stand-by.*
Carrots.
Sun-dried tomatoes in olive oil: *once a luxury, these can now be bought quite inexpensively in many supermarkets. Use them quickly since they don't keep well.*
A red and a green bell pepper.
Plenty of tomatoes.
Celery.
Scallions.
Cucumber.

Miscellaneous

Milk.
Small carton of light cream.
Butter.
Natural and Greek yogurts.
Eggs.
Bacon: *buy small amounts at a time and pay attention to the dates on packages.*
Whole lemon.
Fresh parsley.
Hummus, Tsatsiki, Taramasalata: *watch dates.*
Mayonnaise.
Tomato ketchup.
French mustard.
A mixture of relishes: *to accompany hamburgers (see pages 181–83).*
Fresh fruit juices and carbonated mineral water: *to replace commercial soft drinks.*

the freezer

Whole wheat sliced bread *for toasting.*
Whole wheat or granary rolls *for healthy burgers: see pp 181-83.*
Whole wheat pitas.
Homemade garlic baguettes.
Breadcrumbs: *make these next time you have a few slices of stale bread.*
Spinach, puréed or in leaf form.
Corn, whole or kernels.
Green beans.
Peas.
Broccoli.

Stew packages of mixed vegetables: *to form the basis of a quick nourishing soup.*
Stir-fry vegetables: *various combinations available.*
Fish fillets, or other cuts of firm white fish: *can be cooked directly from the freezer.*
Packages of shrimp.
Fish stock: *to make all the difference to a quick fish soup.*
Ready-made shortcrust and filo pastry.
Tomato and other pasta sauces.

Apple purée.
Simple vegetable purées for a young baby.
Summer fruits: *keep a mixture of strawberries, raspberries, blackberries, blueberries.*
Butter.
The family's favorite ice cream.
Selection of herbs.
Whole or ground seeds: *sesame, sunflower, and pumpkin seeds, pine nuts and peanuts; all can be used straight from the freezer.*

kitchen hygiene

Health statistics indicate that food poisoning is an increasingly serious problem. Although there are numerous points on the food chain at which infections can get in, the family kitchen cannot be absolved of all blame for the alarming rise in incidents of food-related illness.

For most healthy adults, a minor bout of food poisoning is an unpleasant inconvenience, but for small children, particularly, or for anyone whose immune system is weakened by illness, an attack of salmonella – just one of the food-poisoning bacteria currently at large – can have very serious consequences.

Throughout the food chain there are places where infection can occur. Intensive food production and the use of antibiotics in animal feed have created many resistant strains of bacteria; the huge expansion of food processing results in more handling with a greater risk of contamination; and the fast-food business is frequently dirty and unhygienic. Every time someone does something to the food you eat there is a risk of contamination – and this includes you cooking in your own kitchen.

Among common hazards in the kitchen are bacteria from uncooked chicken contaminating other food; gravy, stuffing, stews, or ground meat left too long in a warm room or oven; listeria contamination of soft, unpasteurized cheese and pâté (pregnant women should avoid both); poultry and eggs being served undercooked; and shellfish eaten raw or undercooked.

For your children's sake, it is vital to observe the simple rules of hygiene in the kitchen. But, in general, don't be obsessive about cleanliness. In fact, recent studies have suggested that over-clean and germ-free homes, far from protecting children, may actually put them at risk of asthma and other allergic diseases. The reason for this is that their immune systems fail to reach full strength because they do not get enough practice at coping with bugs and germs.

basic hygiene for the kitchen

General

Dish cloths, scouring pads, and sponges can harbor bacteria. Wash them thoroughly in hot water after use and replace them regularly. For cleaning surfaces after preparing fish or meat, always use disposable paper towels rather than a dish cloth.

While shopping

• Do not take chilled or frozen food on a long shopping trip. Use an insulated cold storage bag, or buy such items last of all and get them into your own refrigerator or freezer as soon as possible.

• Do not leave chilled or frozen raw meat, poultry, or seafood in a closed car.

Storing food

- Keep cooked foods at the top of the refrigerator and raw meat, poultry, and fish at the bottom.
- Never put cooked food on a plate or dish which previously held raw poultry, fish, or meat.
- If your refrigerator does not have a built-in temperature gauge, buy a thermometer and make sure it is always between 32°F and 40°F. Get another for your freezer and keep it below −20°F.
- Make sure you remove all stuffing from cooked chicken or turkey before storing it in the refrigerator. It is actually better to cook stuffing separately if you anticipate having leftovers.
- Cover cooked food and cool it as quickly as possible; refrigerate it within two hours.
- Put leftovers in several smaller containers for more rapid cooling in the refrigerator.
- Do not overfill your refrigerator: it is the circulating air inside that keeps your food safely at the right temperature.

Preparing food

- Wash your hands with warm soapy water and dry them on paper towels before and between handling different foods.
- Wash all fruit, vegetables, and salad ingredients, even prepacked and prewashed ones.
- Wash knives, chopping boards, and counter tops with hot soapy water after use.
- Do not use the same knives and chopping boards for raw and cooked foods.
- Never allow pets onto kitchen work surfaces or to eat off plates or bowls used by the family.

Safe cooking

- Cook all poultry and burgers completely until there are no pink areas.
- Use a meat thermometer. Cook roasts and steaks to at least 290°F, whole chickens or turkey to 360°F, and burgers to 320°F. If you're eating out, break open children's burgers and do not let them eat them if they are still pink. It is safe to eat underdone steak or roasts – minimum 290°F – since any bacteria will be on the outside, which gets much hotter. When meat is ground any bacteria inside are spread throughout the food, so the temperature must reach at least 320°F to destroy them all.

- Cook eggs until they are firm, not runny, unless you know they are organic, or free-range, and free of salmonella. Some supermarkets now sell pasteurized eggs, which can safely be used in homemade mayonnaise.
- Cook fish until it flakes easily with a fork and has turned just opaque.

Frozen foods

- Unless labels on frozen packaged foods say the foods can be cooked directly from the freezer, make sure they are thawed first. Always cook them for at least the time and at the temperature indicated on the package. Frozen poultry should be left to defrost very slowly in the refrigerator. Never try to defrost poultry in hot water.
- Be very careful with microwaves. There may be "cold spots" where bacteria are not killed. If your microwave does not have a turntable, switch it off and turn the dish by hand at least twice during cooking. If the instructions on a package are not clear, or you do not know the wattage of your microwave oven, check with the manufacturer. Burgers, meat, and poultry are the safest to eat when cooked by conventional methods.
- Never re-freeze previously frozen food. Meat, poultry, or fish in the supermarket may have been frozen before reaching the store, and been thawed there. Counter labels should indicate this, so watch out for them when buying.
- Always defrost or marinate food in the refrigerator, never on the kitchen counter at room temperature.

Reheating food

- When reheating soups, gravy, and all sauces, be sure you bring them to a boil. Other leftovers should be reheated to a temperature of 330°F.
- Keep hot food above 145°F until it is served.
- Never reheat food more than once.

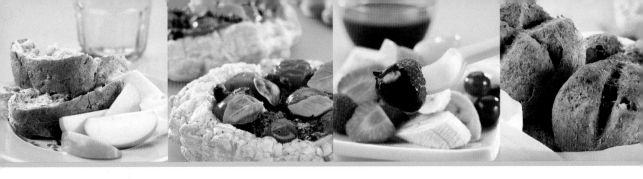

superfood recipes

Here are 160 easy-to-prepare, delicious, and nutritious dishes, all making lavish use of the superfoods in this book. You will find recipes for every meal in a child's day,

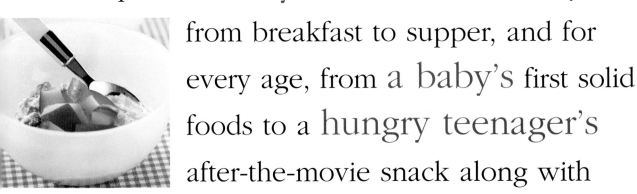

from breakfast to supper, and for every age, from a baby's first solid foods to a hungry teenager's after-the-movie snack along with meals the whole family will enjoy together.

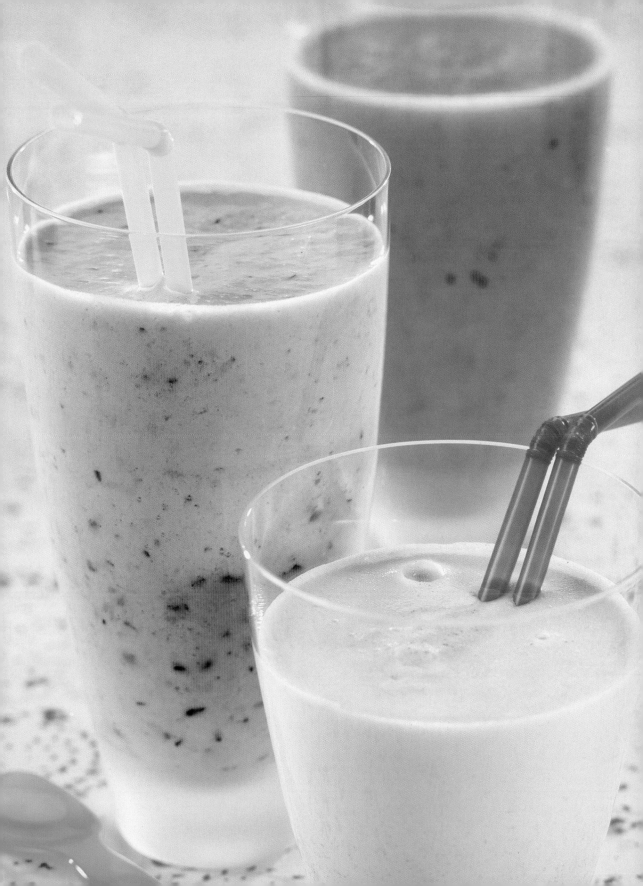

about the recipes

All children are individuals, with their own tastes, appetites, likes and dislikes for food, as much as for everything else. Although every recipe in this book has been carefully planned to use the superfoods in ways that are both nutritious and great to eat, not every child is going to enjoy every one of them.

It is not helpful to establish absolute rules about what foods children will eat, and at what age. It is unrealistic to think that at 4 years and 11 months a child will not like fish cakes and broccoli, yet four weeks later, aged 5, will devour them with relish.

Obviously, there are important guidelines for baby foods, weaning times, and the introduction of solids, and for introducing foods that may potentially be allergens, all of which are included in this book. These excepted, why make your life difficult and your child's miserable by following totally arbitrary rules on what to feed and when?

Every recipe in this book is nutritious, delicious, and healthy. With the exception of babies, for whom specially devised recipes are marked with a symbol (see the box, opposite), all children may happily eat any recipe in this book. If your child's taste is sophisticated and develops in advance of his years, then be happy that you can eat out in interesting restaurants and not be embarrassed by a request for burger and French fries from your 13-year-old.

Even in today's ethnically rich and diverse society, there are still well-meaning but ill-informed health professionals who throw up their hands in horror at the thought of feeding exotic dishes such as curry to small children – a culinary tradition throughout Asia for thousands of years. If a 5-year-old fancies a Vindaloo, let him have it.

What kids should not be offered on a regular basis is the inevitably nutritionally-deficient children's menu familiar in fast food chains, with their litany of burgers and French fries, hot dogs and French fries, chicken nuggets and French fries, fish fingers and French fries, followed by non-dairy ice cream and fruit pie with a soft-drink on the side.

some feeding guidelines

There are a few simple guidelines to bear in mind when feeding children, and you will find them wherever they are relevant in this book. Here is a summary of the most important of them.

• Don't give nuts or anything containing them to children under 5.

• Stick to whole-fat milk and other dairy products for under-5s, rather than semi-skim or low-fat, which do not contain the full complement of the essential fats children need.

• Vary the types of starch – rice, oats, millet, buckwheat, amaranth, spelt, quinoa – that you give your children. Don't feed them wheat more than four times a day.

• Feed your children a wide a range of foods as early as possible, and don't give up if a first attempt fails to please.

• Remember that all children, from babies on up, are sociable creatures and enjoy their food most when they eat with the rest of the family.

time-saving tips in the kitchen

• Before you start a recipe, read it through, and make sure that you have all the ingredients and any necessary equipment on hand.

• Have plenty of paper towels handy to blot meat, fish, and vegetables dry after cleaning them, to drain excess fat from fried foods, to wipe out frying pans, and to mop up spills.

• Clutter slows down cooking: discard waste into the garbage can as you work.

• Make a supply of salad dressing and store it for up to three days in a tightly sealed jar – one with a screw-on lid is ideal – in a cool dark place. It will double as a marinade for chicken and fish.

• Here is how to have a dish to serve pasta in piping hot, without having to use the oven. Place a colander in the serving dish in the sink. When the pasta is cooked, drain it into the colander, pick up the colander, and set it over the saucepan to allow it to finish draining. Tip the hot pasta water out of the serving dish and wipe the dish dry.

• To peel tomatoes and peaches, put them in a bowl and cover with boiling water. Test the skin of one with the tip of a knife and when it is ready to slide off, empty the bowl.

• To peel a clove of garlic quickly, crush it under the blade of a knife.

• Keep a few small bottles containing olive oil, to which you can add a variety of herbs and spices. This way you have homemade flavored oils on hand, like garlic and chilies for a Mexican marinade, rosemary and tarragon for chicken dishes, dill for fish, and oregano for a Mediterranean flavor.

• Keep a shopping list in a prominent place on which to note essential pantry items that are running low, so that you can replace them before they run out.

freezing hints

Although most of the recipes in this book have been devised so that they may be quickly prepared, cooked, and served, they may be frozen in the usual way, if their ingredients allow. The freezer is, in fact, one of your best time-saving assets in the kitchen. For instance:

• Freeze servings of baby food by cooling freshly made purées to room temperature and freezing them in sterilized ice-cube trays. When frozen, transfer the cubes to a freezer bag, label and date and return to the freezer. Use the cubes as required.

• Make large batches of favorite meat-free burgers (see pages 182-84 for recipes) and freeze them. Cool the prepared burgers in the refrigerator for 30 minutes then freeze in a freezer bag, separated by waxed paper. The burgers can be cooked direct from the freezer, allowing extra time to guarantee they are cooked right through. Don't freeze meat burgers: unless they are properly defrosted and cooked completely, they could be a health hazard.

• Parsley, one of the most often used herbs in the kitchen, freezes well. Finely chop a large quantity in the food processor and freeze it. You can then use a little at a time.

• Remove the crusts from whole wheat bread that is beginning to go stale and turn it into crumbs in the food processor. Store the crumbs in the freezer in a lidded carton and use them for croquettes and burgers, or for coating fish.

recipe points to remember

• All spoon measures are level unless otherwise stated. 1tsp = 5ml, 1 tbsp = 15ml.

• Eggs are large.

• Follow either American Standard or metric measurments; don't mix the two.

• Baking times are a guide only, because oven temperatures vary. Use an oven thermometer to check accuracy.

This symbol appears by recipes suitable for giving to babies. The figures with the symbol indicate the age at which the baby may be first offered the food.

big breakfasts

A **great breakfast** is the best way for children to **start** their day. These recipes are packed with **energy** and **essential nutrients**. They look and taste good, too – making the **perfect foundation** for a great day.

muesli

★ = superfood

Serves 2

This simple breakfast recipe is a wonderful source of energy, minerals, and B vitamins.

• Prepare the muesli the night before, making it in individual bowls. For each serving of muesli, stir in enough fruit juice to moisten it well. Then stir in the yogurt and honey. Leave the bowls in the refrigerator overnight.

• In the morning, take the muesli out of the refrigerator as early as possible. Just before it is to be served, stir in fruit of your children's choice of fruit – grated apple or pear, sliced banana, a few strawberries, or a sliced peach. At the Bircher-Benner Clinic in Switzerland, where muesli originated, they add fresh blackberries and some cream.

**2 tbsp organic
unsweetened muesli**
fruit juice, to moisten
★ **2 tbsp natural yogurt**
2 tsp honey
★ **fresh fruit, to serve**

Illustrated right

banana cereal

Serves 1

6 months +

This cereal recipe provides an excellent intake of energy, minerals, and B vitamins and is easily adapted to suit small babies as well as older children.

• For 8–9 month-old babies, or older, use oats straight from the package and add the golden raisins. For babies over 6 months, grind the oats to a fine meal in a clean coffee grinder or a mortar and pestle.

• Put the oats and golden raisins or oatmeal in a saucepan with 2–3 tablespoons of water, breast or organic-formula milk, or a mixture of the two. Bring gently to a boil, reduce the heat, and simmer, stirring occasionally to prevent it sticking, until it has cooked. Mix the banana into the cooked cereal.

★ **1 tbsp organic steel-cut oats**
★ **1 tsp organic golden raisins,
washed (for babies older than
6 months)**
water or milk, to mix (see method)
★ **½ ripe banana, mashed**

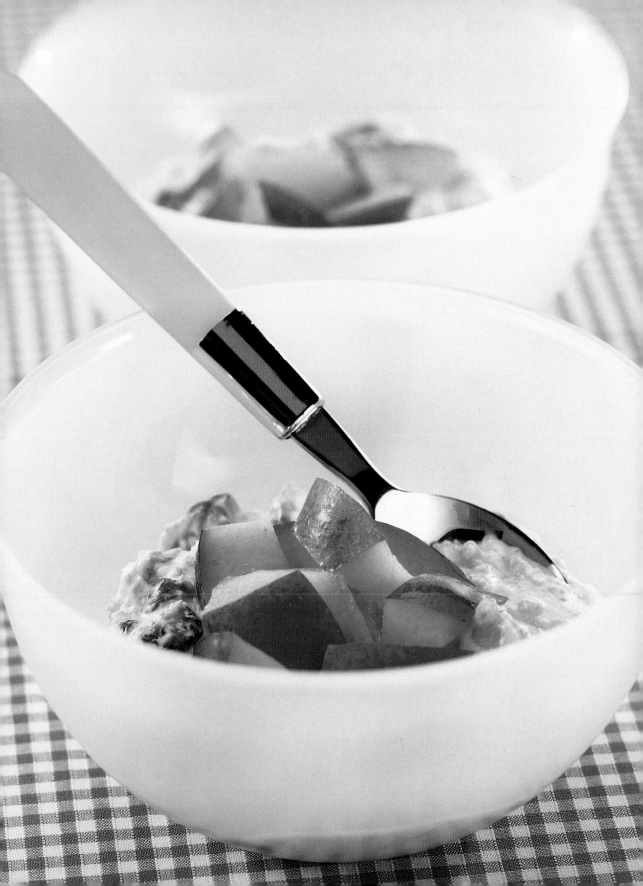

cooked cereal

★ = superfood

Serves 2

Eaten by generations of Scots, cereal is traditionally made with oatmeal, rather than the whole flakes or rolled oats of today's cereal.

- Bring the water to a boil and sift in the oatmeal slowly, stirring all the time, until the water returns to a boil. Lower the heat, cover the pan, and let the oatmeal cook very gently for 10 minutes. Add the salt, stir again and cook for another 10 minutes.
- Add a sweetener before serving, if you like, but remember Scots heroes ate their cereal unsweetened, dipping each spoonful in thick cream.
- Serve with milk or cream, or, if you prefer, with soy or oat milk, or a nut milk made from almonds or hazelnuts (see page 44).

2 cups/500ml water
★ ½ cup/60g medium oatmeal
pinch of salt
honey, maple syrup, or dark brown cane sugar (optional)
★ milk or cream, to serve

other ideas for cereal

- With raisins, honey, and cinnamon. Cook as above, omitting the salt. After 20 minutes, remove from the heat and stir in 2 teaspoons raisins, 1 teaspoon honey, and a pinch of cinnamon. Let stand, covered, for 5 minutes before serving.
- With fruit spread. Instead of sugar, syrup or honey, stir in a spoonful of one of the sugar-free fruit spreads, made with fruit juice concentrates instead of sugar.
- With apple and golden raisins. Cook the oatmeal as above. After 20 minutes, stir in 1 tablespoon peeled and freshly grated apple and a sprinkle of golden raisins.
- Overnight cereal. Heat a wide-mouthed vacuum flask by filling it with hot water then emptying it out. Put in 6oz/180g steel-cut oats, fill with boiling water, close, and leave overnight. At breakfast, the cereal will be ready to eat and still hot. If it is too thick, thin with hot milk or water.

five-grain kruska

Serves 4

This healthy cereal dish, crammed with nutritional riches, appeared in the first *Superfoods* over 10 years ago. A real superfood for hungry, growing children, it was made famous in his own country by the great Swedish naturopath Are Waerland, and popularized in the US by another famous Swedish naturopath, Paavo Airola. The grains should all be organically produced: a filling dish for breakfast or supper.

• Put the whole wheat grains and the millet, oats, rye, and barley in a clean coffee grinder or food processor and process until coarsely ground. Put them in a flameproof casserole, pour in the water, and let them soak overnight.

• In the morning, preheat the oven to 300°F/150°C. Bring the mixture in the casserole to a boil, add the wheatgerm or oatgerm and bran, and the raisins.

• Transfer the casserole to the oven and bake for 30 minutes. The texture should be thick, but not sticky. If it is too thick, add a little more hot water. Serve the Kruska with hot or cold milk, or cream, and a little honey, if desired.

★ 1 tbsp whole wheat berries
★ 1 tbsp whole millet
★ 1 tbsp whole oats
★ 1 tbsp whole rye
★ 1 tbsp whole barley
1 cup/250ml hot water
★ 1 tbsp wheatgerm or oatgerm
★ 1 tbsp wheat or oat bran
★ 2 tbsp raisins or golden raisins
milk or cream, to serve
honey (optional)

creamy yogurt with nuts & honey

Serves 1

Stir the nuts (see page 44) and honey into the yogurt. Greek yogurt provides a nourishing, delicious, and protein-packed start to the day.

★ ½ cup/100g Greek or thick-set natural yogurt
★ 2 tbsp/30g mixed chopped nuts
2 tsp honey

real fruity yogurt

Serves 2

Stir the fruit into the yogurt for a fast and healthy breakfast.

★ ½ cup/100g Greek or thick-set natural yogurt
★ ½ cup/100g whole raspberries, sliced strawberries, peaches, nectarines, or other favorite fruit in season

breakfasts in a mug

★ = superfood

With the best intentions in the world, a leisurely sit-down breakfast isn't always possible. Here are two nourishing protein- and energy-rich breakfasts which can be quickly whipped up in your blender.

banana-to-go

Serves 1

Put the ingredients in a blender and whizz to a deliciously creamy froth.

★ ½ cup/100g natural yogurt
★ 1 banana, sliced
2 tsp brewers' yeast
1 tsp honey

lime-e-shake

Serves 1

Put all the ingredients in a blender (including any citrus-fruit pith saved from the juicer). Blend together well.

★ juice of 2 oranges
juice of 1 lime
★ 1 banana, peeled
★ 1¼ cups/300ml milk
★ ⅔ cup/150g natural yogurt
★ 2 heaping tbsp wheatgerm

apple and apricot purée

Serves 1

4-6 months

• Put the prepared fruit in a saucepan with enough water to cover. Bring to a boil, reduce the heat, and simmer 8–10 minutes, until thoroughly cooked.
• Strain, reserving the cooking water. Purée the fruit, either in a blender or through a strainer. Mix it to a suitable consistency with the reserved water, cooled boiled water, breast milk, or organic formula milk.

★ 1 organic apple, peeled, cored and chopped
★ 2 organic apricots, stones removed

fruitfast

Serves 4

• Wash the fruit thoroughly and drain it well. Put it in a bowl and pour the boiling water over it. Add the orange peel and cinnamon stick, cover the bowl and let it stand overnight.
• The next day, remove the orange peel and cinnamon stick from the fruit and discard. Put a heaping spoonful of thick yogurt on each bowlful before serving.

★ 1lb/500g mixed dried fruit – apricots, prunes, apples, pears, raisins
2½ cups/1.2 liters boiling water
★ a curl of orange peel
★ 3in/7cm piece cinnamon stick
★ thick natural yogurt, to serve

scrambled egg with tomatoes & mushrooms

Serves 1

• Line a broiler pan with foil and heat it. Cut the tomato in half and brush both halves and the mushroom with oil. Put the tomato halves, cut side up, and the mushroom, gill side up, in the broiler pan and broil them until browned, turning the mushroom once during cooking.

• Meanwhile, beat the egg and season it lightly. Put the butter in a small non-stick saucepan and melt it until hot. Add the egg and stir over a high heat until scrambled. Serve with the broiled tomato and mushroom along with whole wheat toast on the side.

★ 1 medium tomato
1 large cremini mushroom
★ a little olive oil
★ 1 egg
salt and black pepper
★ 1 tsp of butter
★ whole wheat toast, to serve

baked eggs & bacon

Serves 6

• Preheat the oven to 350°F/180°C. Use all but 2 tablespoons of the butter to grease six ramekins, each about ⅔ cup/150ml capacity. Put the buttered ramekins in a roasting pan.

• Heat the remaining butter in a small frying pan. Add the bacon pieces and fry them over a medium heat until lightly browned and crisp. Drain the bacon on paper towels, crush the pieces, and sprinkle over the bottoms of the ramekins. Add the parsley and a little seasoning. Break an egg into each ramekin.

• Pour enough hot water into the roasting pan to come halfway up the sides of the ramekins. Cover the pan with foil and bake in the oven for 16–18 minutes until the whites of the eggs are set and the yolks are creamy.

• Spoon some cream over each baked egg and serve immediately with strips of buttered toast.

★ 4 tbsp/60g butter
★ 6oz/180g bacon, chopped
★ 6oz/180g fresh parsley, finely chopped
salt and black pepper
★ 6 eggs
★ ½ cup/100ml heavy cream
★ whole wheat toast, to serve

poached egg & tomato

★ = superfood

Serves 1

In this recipe, the unshelled egg is given an initial dip in boiling water. This sets the egg white slightly so it stays in one piece as it is poaching.

- Bring a small saucepan of water to a rolling boil. Put in the tomato. Put the unshelled egg on a slotted spoon and lower it into the boiling water for half a minute. Lift it out of the water, crack it open, and slide the egg back into the water.
- Poach for 4 minutes, when the tomato and egg will both be done. Lift them out of the pan with a slotted spoon. Serve with buttered whole wheat toast.

★ 1 medium tomato
★ 1 egg
★ whole wheat toast, to serve

french toast

Serves 1

- Melt the butter in a frying pan. Dip the strips of bread in the beaten egg. Put them in the frying pan and fry on both sides until golden.
- Remove the toasts from the pan, sprinkle with a little dark brown sugar and cinnamon and serve while still warm.

★ 2 tbsp/30g butter
★ 1 thick slice whole wheat bread, cut into strips
★ 1 egg, beaten
dark brown sugar, to sprinkle
★ cinnamon, to sprinkle

multi-grain pancakes

Makes 12–16

- Put the dry ingredients, baking powder, baking soda, and salt in a large bowl. Mix well together.
- In a separate bowl, whisk together the eggs, buttermilk, honey, and melted butter. Add the liquid ingredients to the dry ingredients and mix until just combined. (If you overmix the batter the pancakes will be tough; a few lumps are okay.) Gently stir in the toasted pecan pieces.
- Heat a griddle or shallow frying pan over medium-high heat until a drop of water sprinkled on it sizzles. Pour the batter in scant half cupfuls onto the pan and cook for 2–3 minutes until the bubbles form on the surface. Flip each pancake and cook the other side until golden brown. Repeat with the remaining batter. The mixture should make 12–16 pancakes.

★ 3¼ cups/400g dry ingredients, made up of a mixture of cornmeal, rolled oats, whole wheat flour, rye flour, wheat bran, and flax seeds
1 tbsp baking powder
1½ tsp baking soda
½ tsp salt
★ 3 eggs
★ 3 cups/750ml buttermilk
⅔ cup/150g honey
★ 8 tbsp//4oz unsalted butter, melted and cooled
1 cup/125g pecan pieces, toasted

barley cakes

These Scottish pancakes are traditionally cooked on an iron griddle. If you do not have one, use a shallow-sided frying pan or a crêpe pan instead.

• Sift the flour into a bowl. Make a well in the center and break in the eggs. Add the melted butter. Beat the ingredients together, adding enough water to make a smooth batter. Set the batter aside to rest for 30 minutes.

• Heat a griddle or shallow frying pan to moderately hot. Pour a ladleful of the batter on to the heated pan, tilting it so the batter spreads to the edges. Cook for 2–3 minutes, then flip the pancake over and cook on the other side for another 2–3 minutes. Repeat until the mixture is finished. The mixture will make about six cakes.

• When each pancake is cooked, place a filling in the center, fold into quarters and serve while still hot. Good fillings include apple purée; a purée of soaked dried prunes and apricots; a spoonful of berries, such as raspberries, blackberries, or strawberries, stewed over a low heat for 2 minutes, until their juices flow; yogurt with raisins; slices of banana and yogurt; and blackberry jam and Greek yogurt.

★ 1 cup/125g barley flour
★ 3 eggs
★ 2 tbsp/30g butter, melted
water, to mix

oatmeal bannocks (griddle cakes)

• Put the ground oats, salt, and sugar in a large bowl. Dissolve the syrup in the milk and add the mixture to the oatmeal. Cover and let soak overnight.

• The next day, preheat a griddle or shallow frying pan to fairly hot. Mix the eggs and baking soda into the oatmeal. Mix in more milk, if necessary, to make a thick, creamy batter.

• Drop the batter a tablespoonful at a time on to the hot pan – the batter should spread to 5–6 in/12–15 cm. Cook for 2–3 minutes, flip over and cook on the other side for 2–3 minutes.

• As you cook the cakes, pile them on top of one another and wrap in a cloth to keep soft. The mixture should give about 20. Serve them hot with butter and jam.

★ 4 cups/375g old-fashion oats, ground to a coarse flour in a coffee mill
1 tsp salt
1 tbsp sugar
1 tbsp corn syrup
★ 2½ cups/600ml milk
★ 2 eggs, lightly beaten
1 tsp baking soda

super soups

Making soup at home is a fun activity that children enjoy helping with. The results are wonderfully **satisfying**: hot or cold, thick and chunky, or smooth and creamy, soups are **full of goodness** and a pleasure to eat.

minestrone

★ = superfood

Serves 6

This hearty Italian soup is a meal in itself, served with crusty bread and some sticks of fresh carrots and celery to nibble while waiting for it. Minestrone tastes even better the day after it is made.

• Heat the olive oil in a heavy-bottomed saucepan. Add the bacon and fry until it just begins to become translucent. Remove from the pan and set aside. Add the garlic and onion to the pan and fry gently until soft. Return the bacon to the pan with the tomatoes.

• Pour in the hot stock, stir, then add the carrots, turnip, zucchini, celery, and potatoes. Bring to a boil, cover the pan, lower the heat, and simmer very gently for about 40 minutes until the vegetables are tender.

• Add the drained beans and frozen peas and heat through. Add the parsley and seasoning to taste. Serve the soup in warmed bowls, with the Parmesan served separately, to be added according to taste.

★ 1 tbsp olive oil
★ 3 strips of bacon, chopped
★ 1 clove garlic, finely chopped
★ 1 small onion, finely chopped
★ 1 cup/200g canned chopped tomatoes
★ 1 quart/1 liter hot chicken or vegetable stock
★ 2 carrots, finely diced
★ 1 small turnip, finely diced
2 small zucchini, thinly sliced
★ 1 stick celery, sliced
★ 2 potatoes, diced
★ 14oz/425g canned cannellini beans, drained and rinsed
★ ½ cup/60g fresh or frozen peas
★ 1 tbsp finely chopped fresh parsley
salt and black pepper
★ freshly grated Parmesan cheese, to serve

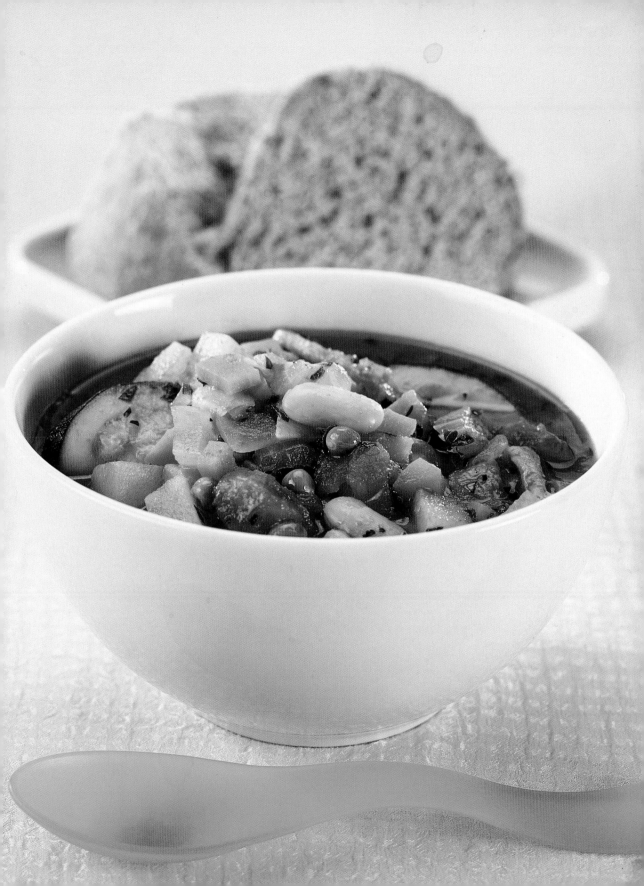

minestrone with pesto

★ = superfood

Serves 6

• Heat the oil in a heavy-bottomed saucepan. Add the onion and garlic, reduce the heat to low, cover the pan, and sweat the vegetables for a few minutes, until translucent. Add the leek, carrot, celery, potato, tomatoes with their juice, and the stock.

• Bring to a boil, reduce the heat, and simmer for about 15 minutes until the vegetables are tender.

• Add the zucchini, cabbage, and a pinch of oregano, and simmer until the cabbage is tender. Add the beans and heat through.

• Taste and adjust the seasoning, if necessary; stir in the pesto sauce, according to taste, and garnish with the torn basil leaves. Serve with Parmesan cheese on the side.

★ 1 tbsp olive oil
★ 1 onion, chopped
★ 2 cloves garlic, chopped
★ 1 leek, sliced
★ 1 carrot, sliced
★ 2 sticks celery, sliced
★ 1 potato, sliced
★ 1 cup/200g canned tomatoes
★ 2½ quarts/1.5 liters chicken or vegetable stock
2 zucchini, sliced
★ ¼ of a small green cabbage, shredded
★ pinch of dried oregano
★ 14oz/425g canned cannellini beans, drained and rinsed
salt and black pepper
pesto sauce, to taste
★ fresh basil, to garnish
★ freshly grated Parmesan cheese, to serve

minestrone with rice & tomatoes

Serves 4

This is a filling summer soup, to be made when tomatoes are cheap and bursting with sunshine. If you use brown rice, allow an extra 20 minutes cooking time.

• Put the tomatoes, onion, and celery in a heavy-bottomed saucepan. Cover the pan and cook over a very low heat until the tomatoes are soft and pulpy.

• Pour the tomato mixture into a food processor or blender and process until smooth. Return the mixture to the pan, add the stock, and bring to a boil. Add the rice. Cover the pan and cook over a very low heat for about 15 minutes, or until the rice is tender.

• Stir in the butter, add a little pepper, and either sprinkle with the chopped basil or stir in the pesto. Serve sprinkled with the grated Parmesan cheese.

★ 1 lb/500g tomatoes, peeled and chopped
★ 1 small onion, roughly chopped
★ 1 stick celery, roughly chopped
1 quart/1 liter vegetable stock
★ ½ cup/100g long-grain rice
★ 2 tbsp/30g butter
black pepper
★ bunch of fresh basil or 2 tsp pesto sauce
★ 2 tbsp freshly grated Parmesan cheese, to garnish

high-protein tofu broth

Serves 4

• Heat the stock in a heavy-bottomed saucepan and add all the remaining ingredients, except the cilantro. Bring to a boil, reduce the heat, cover the pan, and simmer for about 10 minutes, or until all the vegetables are tender.

• Serve the broth immediately, sprinkled with the freshly chopped cilantro.

Note: Tamari sauce, a Japanese variety of soy sauce, is available from ethnic and health food stores.

2 cups/450ml vegetable stock
★ 4oz/125g firm tofu, cubed
★ 1 large carrot, very thinly sliced
★ 2 scallions, chopped
★ white part of 1 small leek, thinly sliced
★ 1 tbsp organic tamari sauce or dark soy sauce
black pepper
★ small bunch cilantro, chopped

leek & watercress soup

Serves 4

• Melt the butter in a heavy-bottomed pan. Add the leek and cook gently until soft. Add the potatoes and stir them in the butter for 1–2 minutes. Add the water, bring to a boil, cover the pan, and simmer for 10 minutes until the potatoes are cooked.

• Meanwhile, discard the thickest stems of the watercress, saving a couple of sprigs for garnish, and finely chop the rest. Add to the soup when the potatoes are almost done and simmer 1–2 minutes.

• Cool slightly then pour into a food processor or blender and process very lightly. Return to the pan and heat through, check the seasoning, swirl in the cream, and garnish with the watercress sprigs.

★ 4 tbsp/60g butter
★ 1 leek, trimmed and finely sliced
★ 2-3 potatoes, unpeeled, sliced
1 quart/900ml water
★ 1 bunch watercress, thoroughly washed
salt and black pepper
★ 2 tbsp cream

creamy celery soup

Serves 4

• Chop the knobbly skin off the celeriac, slice the flesh, and drop it into a bowl of water with the lemon juice or vinegar (to prevent the celeriac discoloring).

• Melt the butter in a saucepan. Add the onion, sweat it for 1–2 minutes, then add the celery, drained celeriac, and potato. Add the stock, bring to a boil, reduce the heat, cover, and simmer for 25–30 minutes, or until the vegetables are tender.

• Pour the soup into a food processor or blender and process briefly, then return it to the pan or a serving bowl. Just before serving the soup, beat the egg yolk into the cream and whisk the mixture into the soup; do not reheat it. Sprinkle with the celery tops, or with chives or parsley before serving.

★ 1 small celeriac root
1 tbsp lemon juice or white wine vinegar
★ 2 tbsp/30g butter
★ 1 onion, chopped
★ 4 sticks celery, sliced; feathery tops reserved for garnish
★ 1 small potato, diced
★ 1 quart/900ml chicken or vegetable stock
★ 1 egg yolk
★ 3 tbsp cream or crème fraîche
★ 1 tbsp chopped fresh chives or parsley, to garnish (optional)

beets & apple soup

★ = superfood

Serves 4

This beautiful red, sweet, and slightly earthy soup is delicious served with plenty of crusty bread.
- Put the beets and onion in a food processor or blender. Add a cupful of the apple juice and process until you have a smooth purée. Stir in the rest of the apple juice and the lemon juice. Add a pinch of sea salt and black pepper.
- Chill the soup for 1–2 hours. Serve it in individual bowls, swirling in the cream just before serving.

★ 1lb/500g raw beets, grated
★ 1 small onion, finely chopped
★ 2½ cups/600ml unsweetened apple juice
★ 1 tsp lemon juice
sea salt and freshly ground black pepper
★ ⅔ cup/150ml sour cream or light cream

baked savoy cabbage soup with melted cheese

Serves 6

This warming soup is more like a casserole and will serve a family of six for a weekend lunch. The best cheese to use is Italian fontina, but a medium Cheddar, Havarti, Gruyère, or Emmenthal would also be delicious.
- Preheat the oven to 400°F/200°C. Heat 2 tablespoons of the olive oil in a large flameproof casserole. Add the garlic and fry gently until just soft. Remove the garlic with a slotted spoon and set aside. Cut the bread into slices 1in/2.5cm thick. Add the remaining oil to the casserole and heat until hot. Add the bread slices in batches and fry until light golden on each side. Remove and reserve.
- Heat the stock in a separate pan and add the cabbage. Bring to a boil, reduce the heat, and simmer for about five minutes until the cabbage is just tender. Drain the cabbage, reserving the stock.
- To assemble the soup, lay some slices of fried bread across the bottom of the casserole. Sprinkle with some garlic, spoon a layer of cabbage on top, dot over a few of the anchovies, then add a handful of the grated cheese, evenly spread. Continue with the same layering until everything is used, finishing with a layer of cheese. Spoon over all the reserved cabbage stock.
- Bake in the oven for about 30–40 minutes, or until a golden crust is formed. Serve in warmed shallow soup bowls, garnished with a little parsley.

★ 4 tbsp olive oil
★ 2 cloves garlic, thinly sliced
1 stale French baguette (approximately 7oz/200g)
★ 1 quart/1 liter chicken stock
★ 1 Savoy cabbage, washed, de-stalked and finely shredded
★ 2oz/60g salted anchovies
★ 7oz/200g grated cheese
★ chopped fresh flat-leafed parsley, to garnish

pumpkin soup

Serves 6

• Remove the skin and seeds from the pumpkin, and cut the flesh into large cubes. Heat the oil in a heavy-bottomed saucepan or flameproof casserole, add the potato, and cook gently until golden but not brown. Add the onion and garlic, mixing them with the diced potato. Add the stock, then the pumpkin, and the sage. Bring to a boil, reduce the heat, cover, and simmer gently for 20–25 minutes until the potatoes and pumpkin are both soft.

• Pour the mixture into a food processor or blender and process to a smooth purée. Return to the pan and heat through. Swirl in the crème fraîche and spoon the soup into bowls. Sprinkle the grated cheese on top, and serve the croûtons separately.

★ 1 pumpkin, weighing about 1 kg/2lb
★ 2 tbsp olive oil
★ 1 small potato, diced
★ 1 onion, chopped
★ 1 clove garlic
1 quart/900ml vegetable stock
★ 4 fresh sage leaves, chopped
★ ⅔ cup/150ml crème fraîche
2oz/60g Gruyère cheese, grated
croûtons, to serve

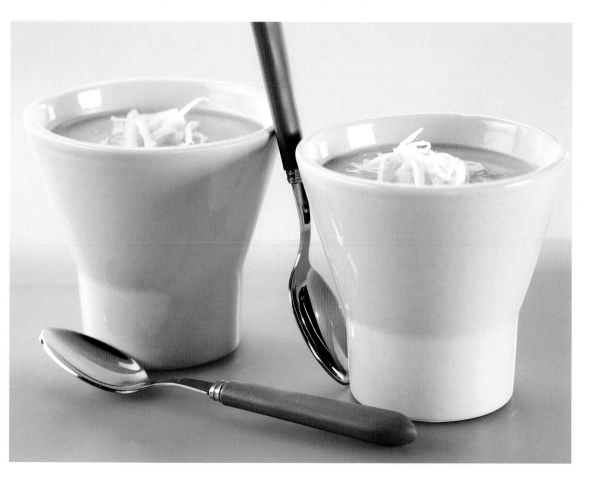

split pea & rice soup

Serves 4

• Rinse and drain the split peas. Put them in a heavy-bottomed saucepan with the water. Bring to a boil, reduce the heat, cover, and simmer for 1 hour.
• When the split peas are nearly cooked, heat the oil in another heavy-bottomed saucepan or a flameproof casserole. Add the onions and garlic and stir-fry until softened but not browned. Add the cumin and stir-fry for a few minutes more.
• Drain the split peas and return them to the pan. Add the onion mixture, vegetable stock, lemon juice and cooked rice. Heat through and season with the pepper. Serve the soup in individual warmed bowls garnished with the chopped cilantro.

★ = superfood

★ 2 cups/250g split peas
1 quart/1 liter water
★ 2 tbsp olive oil
★ 2 large onions, chopped
★ 1 clove garlic, crushed
★ 1 tsp cumin seeds
2 cups/500ml vegetable stock
★ 2 tsp lemon juice
★ a heaping tbsp cooked brown rice
black pepper
★ chopped cilantro

cream of smoked haddock & potato soup

Serves 4

This delicious and substantial winter soup is a favorite on the menu of Zilli's restaurant in London. Try adding some parsnips to the ingredients here, cooking them with the potatoes. Their sweetness will give the soup an enticing flavor.
• Melt the butter in a heavy-bottomed saucepan. Add the onion and cook for 2–3 minutes over a medium heat, until softened but not browned. Stir in the potatoes, reduce the heat and cover the pan tightly. Cook for 10 minutes, stirring frequently, until the potatoes are very tender. Add the haddock to the pan, then stir in the milk and bring to a simmer. Cook for 10–15 minutes until the fish is very tender.
• Pour the soup into a blender or food processor and process until completely smooth. Pour back into the pan, add half the parsley, and reheat until bubbling. Taste and add seasoning, if necessary.
• Ladle the soup into four warmed bowls and sprinkle with the remaining parsley. Serve immediately with lots of crusty bread.

★ 6 tbsp/90g unsalted butter
★ 1 large onion, finely sliced
★ 4oz/125g potatoes, diced
★ 1lb/500g undyed smoked haddock fillet, skinned, boned and diced
★ 5 cups/1.2 liters milk
★ 6 tbsp chopped fresh flat-leafed parsley
salt and white pepper

fish soup with rouille & croûtons

Serves 4

• Clean and skin the fish, being careful to remove all bones. Cut it into chunks and set aside.

• Heat the oil in a large saucepan. Add the onion, garlic, and leeks and cook them over a gentle heat, stirring from time to time until they are softened but not browned. Add the tomatoes, let them cook a little until their juices run; then add the oregano, a pinch of salt, and a little black pepper. Add the fish, then pour in the stock or stock-and-water mixture. Cover the pan and cook gently for 15–20 minutes, or until the fish is cooked through.

• Meanwhile, make the rouille and croûtons. For the rouille, put the mayonnaise into a bowl and stir in the tomato purée, crushed garlic, and chili powder. For the croûtons, bake the slices of French bread in a moderately hot oven (400°F/200°C) for 20 minutes, then cut them into cubes.

• When the fish is done, pour the contents of the pan into a food processor and blend to a smooth purée. Return the soup to the pan and stir in the crème fraîche. Heat the soup through and serve it sprinkled with chopped parsley, serving the rouille and croûtons in separate bowls.

★ 1lb 7oz/675g white fish
★ 2 tbsp sunflower oil
★ 1 onion, chopped
★ 2 cloves garlic
★ white part of 2 leeks, sliced
★ 3–4 large juicy tomatoes, chopped
★ pinch of dried oregano
  salt and black pepper
★ 5 cups/1.2 liters fish stock or half stock and half water
★ 1 tbsp crème fraîche
★ handful of parsley, finely chopped

For the rouille:

4 tbsp mayonnaise
★ 1 tbsp tomato purée
★ 2 cloves garlic, crushed
good pinch of chili powder

For the croûtons:

4 slices French bread

tasty lunches

At lunchtime, children need **nourishing** food to keep their activity and **concentration levels** high for the rest of the day. Here are great choices from purées for babies to food that will **satisfy** hungry schoolchildren.

root vegetable & potato purée

★ = superfood

Serves 1

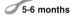 **4-6 months**

You need approximately equal amounts of each vegetable (organic, if possible) for this purée.
• Put the vegetables in a saucepan. Add enough water to cover. Put a lid on the pan, bring to a boil, reduce the heat and simmer gently for about 10 minutes, or until the vegetables are cooked.
• Lift out the vegetables with a slotted spoon, reserving the water. Purée the vegetables in a food processor. Mix the purée to a suitable consistency with some of the reserved water, or with cooled boiled water, breast milk, or organic formula milk.

¼ rutabaga, cut into chunks
1 small parsnip, cut into chunks
★ 1 small potato, peeled and chopped

broccoli, green bean, & sweet potato purée

Serves 1

5-6 months

By the time your baby is 5–6 months old, you can start to introduce green vegetables – ideally, organic.
• Put the chopped sweet potato in a saucepan with enough water to cover. Bring to a boil, reduce the heat, and simmer for 5 minutes. Add the broccoli and beans and cook for another 5–6 minutes until the vegetables are soft.
• Strain the vegetables, reserving the water. Purée the vegetables in a food processor or through a strainer. Mix the purée to a suitable consistency with a little of the reserved water, or with cooled boiled water, breast milk, or organic formula milk.

★ ½ sweet potato, peeled and cut into chunks
★ 3–4 broccoli florets, chopped
★ a few green beans, strings removed and chopped

Illustrated right

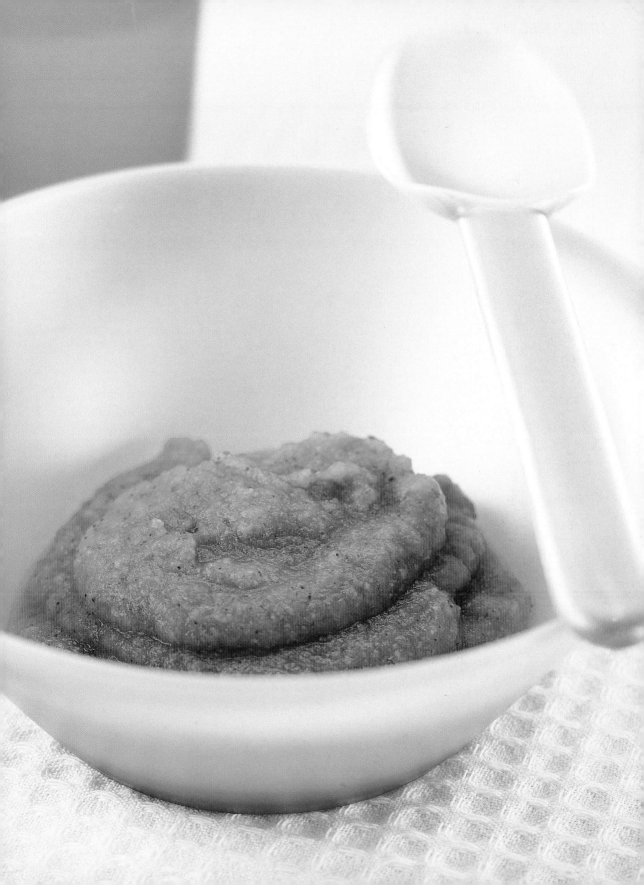

chicken salad with honey & chili

★ = superfood

Serves 4–6

• Beat the egg white and cornstarch together in a bowl. Add one garlic clove and the chicken pieces and stir them so they are well-coated in the egg white. In a separate bowl, mix together the honey, vinegar, soy sauce, and mustard until dissolved. Set aside. Arrange two radicchio leaves on each plate.
• Heat a wok or frying pan and add the oil. When the oil smokes, add the chicken pieces and stir-fry until golden. Remove the chicken from the pan with a slotted spoon and set aside. Add the peanuts to the pan, stir-frying them until golden. Remove from the pan and set aside. Add the chilies (if using), remaining garlic clove, and scallions to the pan. Stir-fry for 1 minute. Put the chicken and nuts back in the pan, add the honey and vinegar mixture and let the sauce bubble a little and reduce.
• Spoon the chicken and sauce over the lettuce and scatter with the tomato halves, and with the cilantro and parsley. Serve immediately.

★ 1 egg white
★ 1 tbsp cornstarch
★ 4 chicken breast halves, skinned, boned, and cut into 2in/5cm pieces
★ 2 garlic cloves, crushed
2 tbsp honey
2 tbsp rice vinegar
★ 2 tbsp soy sauce
1 tsp mustard
★ 8 cup-shaped radicchio lettuce leaves
★ 4 tbsp olive oil
★ 4oz/125g unsalted peanuts (omit for small children)
★ 1-2 tiny dried red chilies (1 or omit for younger children)
★ 12 scallions, trimmed and cut diagonally
★ 12 cherry tomatoes, halved
★ cilantro sprigs
★ flat-leafed parsley sprigs

marinated broiled chicken

Serves 4

Serve these delicious chicken pieces with broiled or steamed vegetables and a garlic mayonnaise.
• Score the chicken breasts two or three times with a sharp knife and place in a baking dish. Mix together the remaining ingredients and pour over the chicken. Chill for at least 2 hours.
• Take the chicken pieces out of the marinade. Lay the herb sprigs over them and either broil under a hot broiler for 8–10 minutes on each side, or bake in a moderately hot oven (400°F/200°C) for 20–25 minutes, or until no pink shows. Baste the chicken pieces occasionally with the marinade. The chicken is done when the juices run clear when the pieces are pierced with a skewer.

★ 4 chicken breast halves
★ juice of 1 lemon
★ 4 sprigs rosemary
★ 4 sprigs thyme
★ 2 cloves garlic, roughly chopped
★ 2 tbsp soy sauce
1 tbsp honey
sea salt and black pepper

fishy feast

Serves 2

This recipe makes enough to feed a hungry toddler and the grown-up who is helping him or her to eat.
• Put the milk into a small saucepan with the herb and lemon zest. Bring to a boil, reduce the heat, and add the fish and potato slices. Simmer for 3–4 minutes, until the fish is cooked. Remove the fish from the pan with a slotted spoon, leaving the potatoes still cooking.
• Skin and flake the fish, being careful to remove all bones. Put the fish into a small buttered casserole. When the potato is cooked, take the pan off the heat and remove and discard the lemon zest. Mash the potato into the milk with a fork and spoon it on top of the fish in the casserole. Sprinkle the wheatgerm over the top, dot with butter, and brown under a broiler.

★ 1¼ cups/300ml milk
★ 1 tbsp chopped fresh mint or parsley
★ a curl of lemon zest
★ 3½oz/100g smoked haddock
★ 2 potatoes, peeled and thinly sliced
★ 1 tsp butter
★ 2 tsp wheatgerm

salmon fish cakes

Makes 4

• Cook the potatoes until soft. Drain, return to the pan they were cooked in, and heat for a few seconds to dry off any residual water. Mash the potatoes with the butter, scallions, and parsley.
• Break the salmon up into small pieces with a fork and mix it into the mashed potato. Add seasoning to taste. If the mixture seems too thick, stir in a little milk. Shape the mixture into four cakes.
• Heat the oil in a frying pan. Add the fish cakes and cook them for a few minutes on each side, until they are brown and crispy. Remove them with a slotted spoon and drain on paper towels. The fish cakes are delicious served hot or cold.

★ 1lb/500g potatoes, peeled and quartered
★ 8 tbsp/125g butter
★ 2 scallions, finely chopped
★ generous handful of fresh parsley, finely chopped
★ 1½lb/750g canned salmon, drained
salt and black pepper
★ ⅔ cup/150ml olive oil

old-fashioned kedgeree

Serves 4

★ = superfood

Use natural (undyed) smoked haddock or cod for this dish. Salmon, smoked salmon, and/or shrimp are also very good additions, especially if you are serving this for a child's main meal of the day.

- Rinse the rice well and drain it well. Put it in a saucepan and pour in a boiling water. Bring the water to a simmer, cover the pan, and cook the rice gently for 35 minutes. Drain, if necessary, and gently fork the rice up to separate the grains.
- While the rice is cooking, cook the fish. Place it in a shallow pan and pour in enough milk to cover. Bring slowly to a boil, then turn off the heat and cover the pan. Do not disturb it for 10 minutes, during which time the fish should be just cooked but still succulent. Lift the fish from the pan with a slotted spoon and skin and flake it, making sure all the bones are removed.
- Stir the fish and the remaining ingredients gently into the warm rice, reserving a few pieces of egg for garnish. The diced butter should melt into it. Taste and adjust the seasoning, if necessary. Serve the kedgeree garnished with the reserved egg and with extra chopped parsley, if desired.

★ 1¼ cups/250g whole-grain long-grain rice
5 cups/1.2 liters lightly salted boiling water
★ 8oz/250g cooked flaked fish
★ milk, to cover
★ 4 hard-boiled eggs, chopped
★ 2 tbsp/30g butter, diced
1 tsp mild curry powder
★ 1 tbsp chopped fresh parsley
★ generous squeeze of lemon juice
sea salt and black pepper
★ 2 tbsp cream (optional)

smoked mackerel quiche

Serves 4

- Heat the oven to 400°F/200°C. Roll out the pastry on a lightly floured surface and use to line an 8in/20cm flan pan.
- Spread the flaked mackerel over the pastry. Scatter the well-drained corn over the mackerel. Whisk the egg lightly in a bowl and add the cream, milk, and seasoning. Whisk again lightly to mix and pour over the mackerel and corn.
- Bake in the oven for about 30 minutes, or until the filling has risen and is golden brown on top.

13oz/400g shortcrust pastry, thawed if frozen
★ 2 smoked mackerel fillets, each about 8oz/250g, flaked
★ 11oz/325g canned corn, drained and rinsed
★ 1 egg
★ ⅔ cup/150ml whipping cream
★ ⅔ cup/150ml milk
pinch salt and black pepper

colcannon

Serves 6

This traditional Irish country dish is comfort food for the coldest days of winter.

• Cook the cabbage in boiling water until tender. Drain and chop it finely and set it aside. Boil the potatoes, carrot, and turnip together in water until tender, then drain them. In a separate pan, simmer the leek and milk together until the leek is tender.

• Add the nutmeg and a little pepper to the potato mixture. Pour the leeks and milk into the potato mixture. Mash all the vegetables well together, adding more milk, if necessary, to make a firm, smooth purée. Add the chopped cabbage and the butter and mash a little more. Pile the mixture into a heatproof dish, rake the top with a fork, and put under a hot broiler to brown.

★ 8oz/250g white cabbage, halved and cored
★ 1lb/500g potatoes, sliced
★ 1 small carrot, diced
★ 1 small turnip, diced
★ 1 small leek, well washed and thinly sliced
★ ½ cup/125ml milk, plus extra for mashing vegetables
★ a pinch of nutmeg
a little black pepper
★ 6 tbsp/90g unsalted butter, diced

vegetable nests with crunchy cheese topping

Serves 4

• First, make the topping. Put the breadcrumbs, flour, seasoning, basil, cornflakes, and grated cheese into a bowl and rub in the butter. Set aside.

• Heat the oil in a large, heavy-bottomed saucepan and add the carrots, zucchini, and parsnip. Fry the vegetables for a few minutes, turning, until golden on all sides.

• Stir in the flour and pour on the vegetable stock. Bring to a simmer, stirring all the time. Stir in the broccoli and cauliflower florets. Simmer very gently for about 15 minutes, until the vegetables are tender. Add the parsley, a little seasoning to taste, and the crème fraîche.

• Transfer the vegetables to an ovenproof dish. Sprinkle on the topping and bake in a moderately hot oven (375°F/190°C) for 30 minutes, or until golden on top.

★ 2 tbsp olive oil
★ 2 carrots, cut into matchsticks
2 zucchini, cut into matchsticks
1 parsnip, cut into matchsticks
1 tbsp flour
1¼ cups/300ml vegetable stock
★ 4oz/125g broccoli florets
★ 4oz/125g cauliflower florets
★ 1 tbsp chopped parsley
salt and black pepper
★ 2 tbsp crème fraîche

For the topping:
2 slices brown bread, crumbed
★ ½ cup/60g whole wheat flour
salt and black pepper
★ 1 tsp dried basil
★ ½ cup/60g cornflakes
★ 2 tbsp Parmesan or Cheddar cheese, finely grated
★ 4 tbsp/60g butter

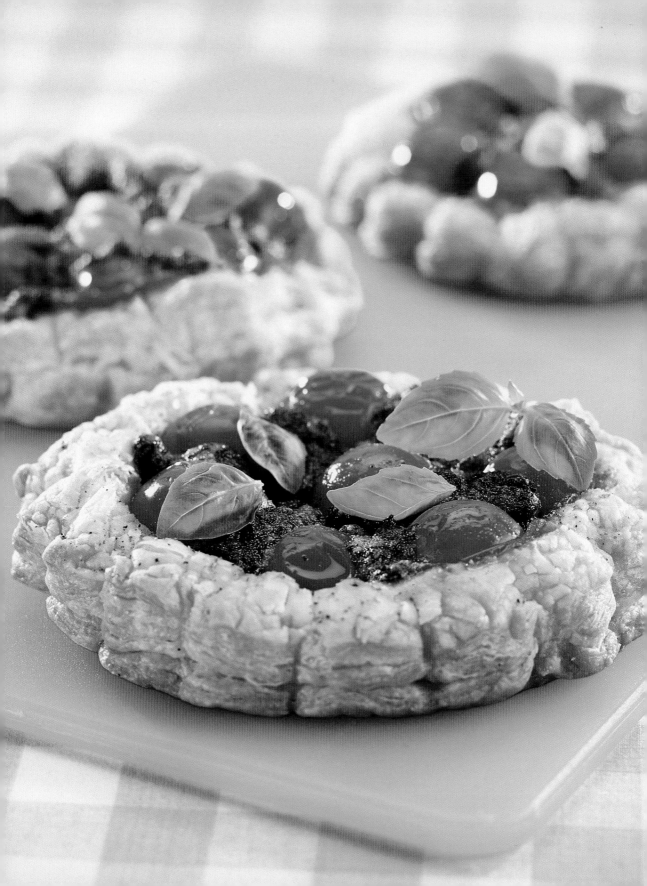

pesto & tomato tarts

★ = superfood

Makes 6

• Preheat the oven to 400°F/200°C. Roll out the puff pastry on a lightly floured surface to a thickness of ¼in/5mm. Cut out six rounds, each about 6in/15cm, using a small bowl or saucer as a guide. Crimp the edges of the rounds with a knife and prick all over with a fork. Put them on a lightly floured baking sheet and bake for 5 minutes. Take the baking pan out of the oven.

• Spread a smooth layer of tomato purée over each pastry round. Lay the cherry tomato halves, flat side down, over the tomato purée. Season with salt and pepper and dot generously with pesto. Drizzle over a little olive oil and return the baking pan to the oven. Bake for a further 10 minutes until the pastry is golden. Serve the tartlets garnished with basil leaves. They are delicious hot or cold.

Illustrated left

12oz/375g puff pastry, thawed if frozen

★ 1¼ cups/300ml tomato purée (strained tomatoes)

★ 6oz/180g cherry tomatoes, halved

3½oz/100g pesto sauce

sea salt and black pepper

★ olive oil, to drizzle

★ fresh basil, to garnish

tomato & cheese bread pudding

Serves 4

• Preheat the oven to 375°F/190°C. Lightly grease a 2 quart/1.8 liter-capacity gratin dish.

• Cut the tomatoes into slices about 5mm/¼in thick, cutting away the central cores when you come across them. Lay half the sliced tomatoes in an even layer in the dish. In a bowl, toss together the breadcrumbs, grated cheese, and a generous amount of seasoning. Sprinkle half this mixture over the tomatoes, cover with the remaining tomato slices, then the rest of the breadcrumb mixture.

• Put the pieces of butter over the top and transfer the dish to the oven. Bake for about 40 minutes, or until bubbling juices are clearly visible and the top is browned. Serve the pudding hot.

★ 2lb/1kg fresh tomatoes

★ ½ cup/60g whole wheat breadcrumbs, made from day-old bread

★ ½ cup/60g Parmesan cheese, freshly grated

salt and black pepper

★ 2 tbsp/30g butter, diced

peppers stuffed with quinoa

★ = superfood

Serves 4

• Wash the quinoa in several changes of water and drain it in a strainer. Put the drained quinoa in a small heavy-bottomed saucepan. Pour in the measured water, bring to a boil, reduce the heat, cover, and cook over the lowest possible heat for 20 minutes. Remove from the heat and leave covered in a warm place for 15 minutes.

• Preheat the oven to 400°F/200°C. Heat the oil in a frying pan. Add the onion and garlic and fry gently for a few minutes, until softened but not browned. Add the quinoa, currants, pine nuts, lemon juice, herbs de provence, a pinch of salt, and a little black pepper. Stir the ingredients together.

• Cut the tops off the peppers and set them aside. Core and seed the peppers carefully. Divide the quinoa mixture among the four peppers and put the tops on them. Pack the peppers into an ovenproof dish just big enough to hold them, and brush them with oil. Stir the tomato purée into ⅔ cup/150ml water and pour in around the peppers.

• Bake in the oven for about 45 minutes, until the peppers are cooked but not too soft. If the dish dries out, add a little more hot water. Serve with tomato sauce and a green salad.

★ 6oz/180g quinoa
2 cups/525ml water
★ 2 tbsp olive oil, plus extra for brushing
★ 1 onion, chopped
★ 2 cloves garlic, crushed
★ 1 tbsp currants
★ 1 tbsp pine nuts
★ 1 tsp lemon juice
pinch of herbs de provence
salt and black pepper
★ 4 large red peppers
★ 1 tbsp tomato purée

pisto

Serves 4

This is the Spanish version of those aromatic dishes of stewed vegetables found all round the Mediterranean. Serve it on its own, with broiled meat, fish, or chicken, or with a beaten egg stirred in and cooked for a few minutes more.

• Heat the oil in a heavy-bottomed saucepan. Add the onion, pepper, and garlic and fry gently until just soft. Add the eggplant and fry for a few minutes more, turning several times. Add the tomatoes with all their juices, the potato, zucchini, a pinch of salt, and a grinding of pepper.

• Reduce the heat, cover the pan and cook for 20–25 minutes. Remove the lid and, if there is still a lot of liquid left, cook more briskly, uncovered, for a few minutes. Sprinkle with the herbs and serve.

★ 3 tbsp olive oil
★ 1 onion, chopped
★ 1 large red, green, or yellow pepper, cored, seeded and cut into strips
★ 1 clove garlic, crushed
1 eggplant, diced
★ 4 tomatoes, skinned and chopped
★ 1 potato, diced
1 zucchini, sliced
salt and black pepper
★ plenty of chopped fresh herbs, such as parsley, chives, and basil

spanish omelette

Serves 4

You can make this omelette with almost any leftover vegetable; broccoli, peas, asparagus, and green beans are all good. Make it in a small frying pan, as it will come out too thin if made in a large one.

• Heat the olive oil in the frying pan. Add the potato and fry over a moderate heat until just golden. Add the onion and continue cooking gently until soft but not browned. Add the peppers and cook gently for 3–4 minutes, until just soft.

• Add the eggs, season lightly, and turn the heat down – the omelette should cook very slowly. Once it has started to set, give the pan an occasional shake and do nothing else until the edge of the omelette begins to curl away from the pan.

• When reasonably firm but still moist on top – after about 10 minutes – put the pan under a very hot broiler until the surface of the omelette starts to turn golden brown. Serve hot or cold.

★ 2 tbsp olive oil
★ 1 large potato, diced
★ 1 onion, chopped
★ ½ red pepper, cored, seeded, and chopped
★ ½ green pepper, cored, seeded, and chopped
★ 4 eggs, lightly beaten
sea salt and black pepper

fennel with lemon & mixed herbs

Serves 2–3

This herbed fennel is good with fish. The recipe is also a good way of cooking leeks.

• Cut the bottom and top off the fennel, leaving the white bulbous part. Slice across into fairly thin slices. Melt the butter in a large frying pan. Add the fennel and fry it gently for 10–15 minutes, until it is tender and starting to brown slightly. You may have to add a little more butter during cooking. Transfer the cooked fennel to a serving dish.

• Add another teaspoon of butter to the pan. When it has melted add the mixed herbs and lemon juice and swirl the sizzling mixture around the pan. Pour it over the fennel and serve.

1 large bulb fennel
★ 2 tbsp/30g butter
★ 1 tsp dried mixed herbs
★ juice of ½ lemon

broccoli stir-fried with ginger & garlic

★ = superfood

Serves 4

• Cut the thick stalks off the broccoli and peel and slice them. Break the heads into small florets. Heat the vegetable oil in a frying pan or wok until hot.
• When the oil is hot, put the ginger into the pan and stir once. Add the broccoli, salt and garlic. Stir-fry vigorously for 1 minute, or until the broccoli turns bright green. Add the stock. Cover the pan and cook over a high heat for about 1½ minutes. Remove the pan from the heat. Add the sesame oil and stir to mix. Serve immediately.

★ **1–2 large heads of broccoli**
★ **2½ tbsp vegetable oil**
★ **2 thin slices fresh ginger**
1½ tsp salt
★ **3 cloves garlic, lightly crushed**
3 tbsp vegetable stock
★ **1 tsp sesame oil**

broccoli with potatoes

Serves 4

• Peel the potatoes and cut them into chunky dice the same size as the broccoli florets. Heat the oil over a medium heat in a large non-stick frying pan.
• When the oil is hot, put in the asafetida and, a second later, the mustard seeds. As soon as the mustard seeds begin to pop – a matter of seconds – add the green chili and the curry leaves. Stir once, then add the potatoes. Stir-fry for about 4 minutes, or until the potatoes are very lightly browned.
• Sprinkle in a pinch of salt and toss to mix. Add the broccoli and amchar masala. Stir-fry for 1–2 minutes, or until the broccoli is heated through. Remove the chili and serve immediately.

★ **8oz/250g waxy potatoes, boiled, drained and cooled**
★ **3 tbsp peanut oil**
large pinch of asafoetida
½ tsp brown or yellow mustard seeds
★ **1 fresh green chili, tip cut off**
10 fresh curry leaves
salt
★ **12oz/375g broccoli florets, blanched**
1 tsp amchar masala

tuna & bean salad

Serves 4

• Put the cannellini beans in a bowl. Add the tomatoes, cucumber, and scallions, and mix them all well together.
• Mix the oil, lemon juice, salt, and pepper together and stir into the salad. Fork the tuna into the salad. Arrange the hard-boiled egg halves on top, and sprinkle over the finely chopped herbs.

★ **13oz/400g canned cannellini beans, drained and rinsed**
★ **3 tomatoes, peeled and finely chopped**
½ cucumber, peeled and diced
★ **6 scallions, sliced**
★ **6¼ cup/60ml extra-virgin olive oil**
★ **2 tsp lemon juice**
sea salt and black pepper
★ **6½oz/200g canned tuna, drained and flaked**
★ **2 hard-boiled eggs, halved**
★ **a small bunch of parsley and basil, finely chopped**

bread & tomato salad

Serves 4

Use ripe plum tomatoes when they're at their best and most flavorful. This salad only works with coarse homemade whole wheat bread or good country bread and is really good when both the tomatoes and bread are organic.

• Heat the oil in a large, deep frying pan. Add the cubes of bread and the garlic. Fry, stirring continuously, until the bread becomes crisp. Drain the bread cubes on paper towels.

• Put the bread cubes into a bowl, add the chopped tomatoes, lemon juice, the basil, a pinch of salt, and plenty of freshly ground black pepper. Toss all the ingredients together well and serve.

★ 3 tbsp extra-virgin olive oil

4 thick slices of bread, crusts removed and cut into 1in/2.5cm cubes

★ 2 cloves garlic, chopped

★ 6 ripe plum tomatoes, chopped

★ 1 tbsp fresh lemon juice

★ 2 tbsp fresh basil, torn in pieces

salt and black pepper

pasta salad with tuna

Serves 4

• Bring a large pan of water to a boil, add a dash of vegetable oil and 1–2 teaspoons of ordinary salt, then add the pasta.

• While the pasta is cooking, mix the olive oil, lemon juice, mustard, sea salt, and pepper together to make a dressing.

• When the pasta is just tender – it should have a little bite to it – drain it well, and put it into a serving bowl. Pour over the dressing and toss together. Gently mix in the tomatoes, scallions, and tuna, then sprinkle with the parsley.

★ dash of vegetable oil

salt

★ 8oz/250g spiral pasta

★ 2 tbsp extra-virgin olive oil

★ 2 tsp lemon juice

1 tsp Dijon mustard

sea salt and black pepper

★ 3–4 ripe tomatoes, peeled and chopped

★ 6 scallions, sliced

★ 6½oz/200g canned tuna, drained and flaked

★ 1 tbsp chopped fresh parsley

buckwheat crêpes

Makes 12

The best way to serve these crêpes is to put some filling (see below for ideas) on each one, roll it up and enjoy it while it is still warm.

• Stir the melted butter into the milk. Put the flours and salt together in a mixing bowl or into a food-processor bowl. Whisking all the time, pour in the milk-and-butter mixture and then stir in the eggs one at a time, until everything is blended well. Allow the mixture to rest in the refrigerator for at least 30 minutes.

• Brush an 7in/18cm crêpe pan with a little oil. Place the pan over a medium heat. When the oil is smoking, pour a ladleful of batter into the pan and tilt it around until it spread evenly over the crêpe. When the underside is golden, turn it over and cook on the other side for a minute or two.

• Slide the crêpe out of the pan onto paper towels on a warm plate and keep warm while you make the rest of the crêpes. You will need to re-oil the pan between each crêpe. The mixture should make about 12 crêpes.

★ 2 tbsp melted butter
★ 2 cups/450ml milk
★ 1 cup/125g buckwheat flour
1 cup/125g flour, sifted
½ tsp salt
★ 4 eggs
★ vegetable oil, for frying

filling mixtures for crêpes

• Apple slices, walnuts, and raisins, sprinkled with a little cinnamon and brown sugar, and served with fromage frais, fromage blanc, or Greek yogurt.

• Creamy, mild goat cheese, and honey, or strawberries and blueberries, with a little sugar and freshly squeezed lemon juice.

• Savory fillings such as baked beans, sautéed mushrooms, broiled tomatoes, grated cheese, or ratatouille – the list is endless.

pita plus

Serves 4

• Lightly broil the pita breads on one side and split them while still warm. Mix the shredded radishes with the onion and watercress. Add the tuna and toss it into the radish mixture. Stuff the pita breads with the mixture.

• Serve a small dish of mayonnaise on the side. For a tapenade-flavored mayonnaise, add finely chopped black olives, capers, a couple of anchovy fillets, and a squeeze of lemon.

★ 4 large whole wheat or sesame pita breads

1 bunch radishes, very finely shredded

★ 1 small red onion, very finely sliced

★ 1 bunch watercress, washed and sprigs separated

6½oz/200g canned tuna in oil, drained and flaked

mayonnaise, to serve

four dips

Serve these dips with whole wheat breadsticks or hot pita bread, and with raw vegetables, such as sticks of carrot or celery, chunks of cucumber, radishes, cherry tomatoes, and cauliflower florets.

avocado dip

Serves 4

Prepare the tomato and scallions in advance, if desired. Just before you are ready to serve the dip, halve, pit and peel the avocados, and mash the flesh to a soft purée. Add the lime juice, tomato, scallions, and a little salt and pepper.

★ 1 small tomato, finely chopped

★ 2 scallions, finely chopped

★ 2 ripe avocados

★ juice of 1 lime

salt and black pepper

tomato & yogurt dip

Serves 4

Put the yogurt into a bowl and stir in the tomatoes, oil, and herbs – choose from basil, mint, parsley, or chives, or a mixture. Add seasoning to taste.

★ 1 cup/200g natural yogurt

★ 2 ripe, red tomatoes, peeled and finely chopped

★ 2 tsp extra-virgin olive oil

★ 1 tbsp chopped fresh herbs

cream-cheese dip

Serves 4

Combine the cream cheese, yogurt, and olive oil in a bowl, mixing well until smooth. Add the remaining ingredients, stir thoroughly, chill, and serve.

★ 7oz/200g low fat cream cheese

★ 2 tbsp natural yogurt

★ 1 tsp extra-virgin olive oil

★ 1 tbsp chopped red onion

★ 2 tsp finely snipped chives

black pepper

smoky dip

Serves 4

Put the trout fillet and cottage cheese in a food processor and blend briefly. Add the lime juice and a little pepper and blend again. Spoon into a bowl and serve sprinkled with the red pepper.

★ 1 smoked trout fillet, flaked

★ ⅔ cup/150g cottage cheese

★ juice of ½ lime

black pepper

2 tsp finely chopped red pepper

snacks & light meals

Quickly made snacks and tempting light meals are just what children need to boost energy as their busy day at home, nursery, or school slows down. Here is a great selection to choose from.

quick & easy whole wheat bread

★ = superfood

Makes 1 2lb/1kg loaf

Many variations of this wonderful loaf can be made by mixing different flours: try 2 cups/250g all-purpose, cracked wheat, rye, or buckwheat flour and 4 cups/500g whole wheat flour. You can also use chopped walnuts, pumpkin seeds, pine nuts, or poppy seeds.

- Preheat the oven to 400°F/200°C. Lightly oil a 2lb/1kg loaf pan and keep it warm.
- Mix the flour and yeast together in a mixing bowl. Dissolve the oil, sugar or honey, molasses, and salt in the water. Make a well in the center of the flour, pour in the water and add the sunflower seeds (if using). Mix all the ingredients together with a wooden spoon, then knead the dough for 3–4 minutes, until it comes together in a ball without sticking to the sides of the bowl. Add a little flour if the dough seems too sticky, or water if it is dry and crumbly.
- Put the dough into the warm pan, cover with a clean, damp dish towel and let it rise in a warm place for 30–40 minutes, or until the dough has risen to near the top of the pan.
- Transfer the pan to the oven and bake in the center of the oven for 35–40 minutes. The bread will be ready if it sounds hollow when you tap the bottom of the pan. If it doesn't, bake it for another five minutes. Cool in the pan on a wire rack.

★ **6 cups/750g stoneground whole wheat bread flour**

1 pkg/6g instant dried yeast

★ **2 tsp extra-virgin olive oil**

1 tsp molasses, dark brown sugar or honey

½ tsp salt

2½ cups/600ml lukewarm water

★ **1 tbsp sunflower seeds (optional)**

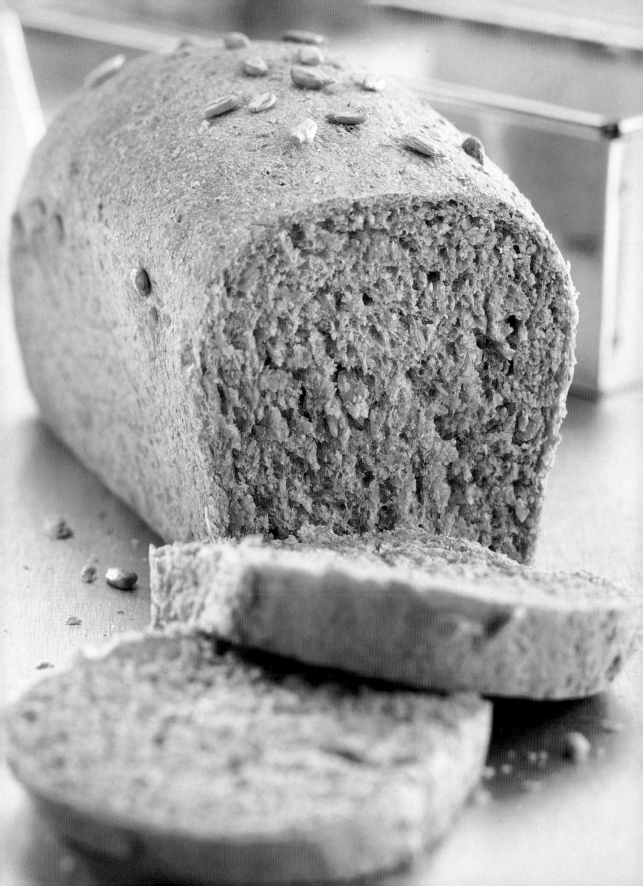

salmon surprise

★ = superfood

Serves 1–2

6-9 months

• Melt the butter in a small non-stick saucepan. Add the onion and cook it over a low heat until it is softened but not browned. Sprinkle the flour over the onion, stirring it in, and add the milk to make a creamy sauce – you may need a little more milk.
• Cook the sauce very gently for about 10 minutes, stirring it occasionally.
• While the sauce is cooking, skin the fish and carefully remove all the bones. Add the fish to the sauce and cook for another 3–4 minutes, or until the fish is tender. Mash the sauce and fish together well.

★ 1 tsp butter
★ ½ small onion, finely chopped
★ ½ tsp whole wheat flour
★ 2 tbsp milk
★ about 2oz/60g salmon fillet

tuna mashed potatoes

Serves 1–2

6-9 months

• Put the potato slices into a saucepan and add enough milk to cover. Add the onion. Bring to a boil, lower the heat, and cook gently until the potatoes are cooked and the milk is almost absorbed. Lightly grease a small ovenproof casserole.
• Mash the potatoes, stirring in the butter, then stir in the tuna. Turn into the casserole, sprinkle the wheatgerm on top, and brown under a hot broiler.

★ 3–6 (depending on size) new potatoes or 2 medium ones, thinly sliced
★ milk, to cover
★ ½ small onion, grated
★ 1 tsp butter
★ 3 tbsp canned tuna
★ 1 tbsp wheatgerm

spinach soufflé

Serves 2

6-9 months

This recipe, like the two above, makes enough to give mother and baby an enoyable light meal.
• Preheat the oven to 375°F/190°C. Lightly butter a small casserole or two ramekins.
• Chop the spinach finely, then mix it with the cottage cheese. Beat the egg yolks lightly; stir the eggs and the grated cheese into the spinach.
• Whisk the egg whites to soft peaks and fold them into the spinach mixture. Spoon the mixture into the prepared dishes. Bake in the oven for 35–40 minutes – a little less if you are using individual ramekins.

★ butter, for greasing
★ 4oz/125g cooked spinach, drained
★ 4 tbsp cottage cheese
★ 2 eggs, separated
★ 2oz/60g grated cheese

fish cakes

Makes 4

- Cook the potatoes in boiling water until soft. Drain them, return to the pan, and heat for a few seconds to dry off any remaining water.
- Put the stock in a saucepan. Add the fish, bring to a boil, reduce the heat, and poach gently for 10 minutes. Drain the fish and flake it very carefully to remove any bones or remaining skin. Mash the potatoes with the butter, chives, and a little salt and white pepper. Mix in the flaked fish. Shape the mixture into four cakes.
- Heat the oil in a shallow frying pan and cook the cakes for a few minutes on each side until brown and crispy. Remove with a slotted spoon and put on paper towels to drain. The fish cakes are delicious served either hot or cold.

★ 1lb/500g potatoes, peeled and quartered
2 cups/900ml vegetable stock
★ 12oz/12oz salmon fillet, skinned
★ 12oz/375g cod fillet, skinned
★ 8 tbsp/125g butter
★ 1 tbsp chopped chives
salt and white pepper
★ ⅔ cup/150ml olive oil

savory egg

Serves 1

- Preheat the oven to 425°F/220°C. Lightly butter a small ramekin.
- Put the chives, grated cheese, and milk into the ramekin. Crack in the egg carefully, in order not to break the yolk. Place the ramekin in a small roasting pan and pour in enough boiling water to come halfway up the side of the ramekin. Bake in the oven for 15–20 minutes, until the egg is set.

★ butter, for greasing
★ chopped chives
★ 1 tsp grated cheese
★ 2 tsp milk
★ 1 egg

mushrooms on toast with crumbly cheese

Serves 2

- Melt the butter in a frying pan. Add the onion, garlic, and mushroom slices and fry them gently until softened. While they are cooking, broil the bacon until crisp.
- Divide the mushrooms between the two slices of the toast and top with the cheese. Put under a hot broiler and broil until the cheese melts. Serve with the crisy bacon slices on top.

★ 2 tbsp/30g butter
★ ¼ medium onion, chopped
★ 1 clove garlic, chopped
4 large flat mushrooms, organic if possible, sliced
★ 8 strips lean bacon
★ 2 slices coarse whole wheat bread, toasted
★ 2oz/60g Cheshire cheese, sliced

quick spinach snack

Serves 2

★ = superfood

It's not always easy to get children to eat spinach, but cooked like this and served as the Italians do – warm rather than hot – you'll be surprised how much they enjoy it, especially if you use superb-tasting organic spinach.

• Heat the oil in a small saucepan. Add the garlic and cook gently for 5 minutes without browning it. Add the pine nuts and cook for another 5 minutes.

• Put the spinach in a large saucepan with no extra water, cover the pan, and cook until thoroughly wilted. Let it cool for a few moments then add the warm oil, garlic, pine nuts, and the lemon juice. Stir well and arrange on top of the bread.

★ 4 tbsp olive oil
★ 1lb/500g young spinach leaves, washed
★ 2 cloves garlic, sliced
★ juice of 1 lemon
★ small handful pine nuts
★ 2 thick slices whole wheat bread

hot pancetta savories

Serves 2–4

• Dry-fry the pancetta in a frying pan until crisp. Drain on paper towels. When cool, mix it with the grated cheese.

• Spread the slices of bread with butter on one side. With the buttered sides facing down, spread the pancetta mixture on top of two slices. Dot with a few basil leaves and press the remaining slices of bread on top, buttered sides facing up.

• Heat the oil in a frying pan. Place the sandwiches in the pan and fry gently for a couple of minutes on each side, or until the cheese is melted and the bread is golden and crisp. Cut the sandwiches into triangles while they are hot and serve immediately.

★ 2oz/60g pancetta, chopped
★ 2oz/60g mozzarella cheese, grated
4 slices whole wheat bread
★ 2 tbsp/30g butter, softened
★ few basil leaves
★ 1 tbsp olive oil

pizza baguettes

Serves 4

Flavored baguettes, such as those made with onion, multigrains, or sun-dried tomatoes, would all taste delicious in this recipe.

• Preheat the oven to 350°F/180°C. Mix the tomatoes, garlic, and basil together and heat gently in a saucepan. Split the baguettes and spread the tomato mixture on the cut surfaces. Drizzle with olive oil, if desired. Sprinkle with grated cheese.

• Bake in the oven for about 10 minutes, or until the cheese has melted and the bread is hot and crisp.

★ 13oz/400g canned chopped tomatoes; or the same weight of fresh tomatoes, skinned and chopped
★ 1 clove garlic, crushed
★ fresh basil leaves
4 baguettes, or the equivalent in lengths of other slim bread
★ olive oil (optional)
★ 4 tbsp grated Cheddar cheese

granny smith's welsh rarebit

Serves 4

Welsh Rarebit is NOT a piece of processed cheese put on a piece of toast and melted under a broiler. Here is a more authentic version.

• Toast the bread and butter it, using about two-thirds of the butter. Keep the toast warm while you make the topping.

• Put the cheese in a heavy-bottomed saucepan and add the crème fraîche and mustard powder. Heat slowly, stirring, until the cheese has melted and the mixture has become a thick cream.

• Melt the remaining butter in a frying pan. Add the apple wedges and fry them gently. Spread the cheese mixture on the slices of toast and brown under a hot broiler. Serve each slice of toast with four wedges of apple.

★ 4 medium-thick slices whole wheat bread
★ 6 tbsp/90g unsalted butter
★ 8oz/250g mature Cheddar cheese, grated
★ 4 tbsp crème fraîche
½ tsp mustard powder
★ 2 large Granny Smith apples, peeled, cored and each cut into 8 wedges

stuffed celery sticks

Serves 2–4

With these ingredients you can give children greens to eat in a way they will enjoy. Simply stuff celery sticks with the following mixtures:

• Cottage cheese with chives: many supermarkets sell this ready-made.

• Grated carrots and raisins tossed in a little oil and lemon juice.

• Grated carrots and shredded watercress mixed into cream cheese.

★ 4–6 sticks celery, trimmed and strings removed
★ cottage cheese with chives
★ carrots, grated
★ raisins
★ vegetable or olive oil
★ lemon juice
★ watercress
★ cream cheese

hummus

Serves 4–6

Hummus is very good served with lots of raw vegetables, such as chicory leaves, sticks of red bell pepper, raw carrots, or celery. It is also great served with hot pita bread, black olives, and whole baked garlic cloves.

• Put all the ingredients, except the olive oil, in a food processor or blender. Switch the machine on and add the olive oil in a steady stream until you have a smooth consistency. The hummus can be thinned with a little of the chickpea liquid, or made more creamy with extra olive oil.

★ **13oz/400g canned chickpeas, drained, or same weight of freshly cooked chickpeas, drained (reserve some of the canning or cooking liquid)**
★ **juice of 1 lemon**
★ **2 cloves garlic, peeled**
★ **2 tbsp tahini (pulped sesame seeds)**
salt and black pepper
★ **½ cup/125ml olive oil**
★ **1 tsp freshly ground cumin**

sandwich fillings

Here are some splendid fillings for sandwiches, using many of the book's superfoods. Make the sandwiches from whole wheat bread, whole wheat pita pockets, or whole wheat rolls.

• Hummus (see above), alfalfa sprouts, chopped tomatoes, and fresh basil or cilantro.
• Peanut butter, bananas, and a little honey.
• Watercress, finely grated carrot, thinly sliced cucumber, and mayonnaise.
• Tuna, thinly chopped celery, and red bell pepper with mayonnaise.
• Shredded chicken, lettuce, chopped tomato, a few bean sprouts, and a few basil leaves, all tossed in a little dressing made with extra virgin olive oil, lemon juice, a pinch of sea salt, and black pepper. Pile this mixture into pita pockets.
• Well-drained canned salmon, sliced scallions, a little chopped fresh parsley, and mayonnaise with half a ripe avocado and a squeeze of fresh lemon juice beaten into it.
• Mashed sardines with paper-thin slices of cucumber and chopped chives.
• Finely chopped apple mixed into smooth peanut butter.
• Cream cheese with shredded lettuce and chopped walnuts.

cheese pretzels

Makes about 20

• Dissolve the yeast and sugar in the warm water. Put the flour, grated cheese, and salt into a food-processor bowl or a mixing bowl. Pour in the water and yeast and mix thoroughly, either by hand or with the dough hook of the food processor.

• Knead the dough in your machine or on a lightly floured surface for 5–10 minutes until smooth and elastic. Cover with a damp cloth and let it rise in a warm place until doubled in size; this should take about 1 hour.

• Punch down the dough and knead it again briefly. Divide it into about 20 pieces and roll into strands. Form the pretzels by looping the strands and twisting over the ends. Place on baking sheets. Let them rise again for about 20–30 minutes. Meanwhile, preheat the oven to 400°F/200°C.

• Brush the risen dough with the egg and sprinkle the seeds on top. Bake in the oven for 20 minutes, until shiny and golden. Cool on wire racks.

1 pkg/6g yeast
1 tsp sugar
1¼ cup/300ml warm water
4 cups/500g all-purpose flour
★ 6oz/180g Cheddar cheese, grated
pinch of salt
★ 1 egg, beaten
★ sesame seeds and poppy seeds, mixed, to sprinkle

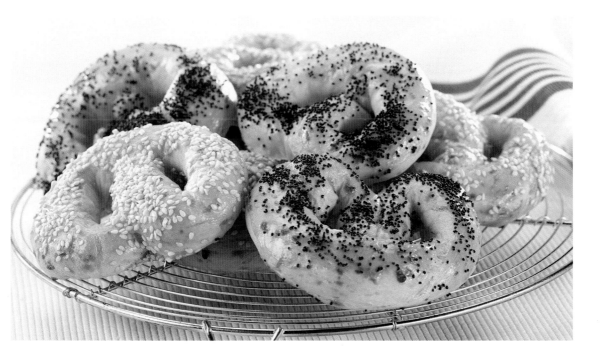

mighty muesli munchies

★ = superfood

Makes 12

• Preheat the oven to 350°F/180°C. Lightly grease a shallow baking pan measuring approximatcly 13 x 10in/33 x 25cm.
• Mix the muesli and spices together in a large bowl. Put the honey, sugar, and butter in a small saucepan and heat slowly until the sugar dissolves. Pour the mixture into the muesli and mix together thoroughly.
• Put half of the muesli mixture in the prepared pan. Mix the bananas, dates, and lemon juice together and spread on top of the muesli mixture. Evenly top it with the rest of the muesli mixture.
• Bake in the preheated oven for 25–30 minutes, or until golden. Let the pan cool. Then cut the mixture lengthwise down the middle and divide each half into six substantial bars.

10oz/300g unsweetened muesli
(preferably without nuts)
★ pinch of nutmeg
★ 1 tsp ground cinnamon
¼ cup/60g honey
½ cup/125g brown sugar
★ 8 tbsp/125g butter
★ 3 ripe bananas, thinly sliced
★ 6oz/180g fresh or semi-dried dates, pitted and chopped
★ juice of 1 lemon

oatcakes

Makes 16

• Preheat the oven to 350°F/180°C. Put the oatmeal in one bowl and the butter and salt in another. Pour the boiling water over the butter and salt. Add this mixture to the oatmeal and mix well. Let it stand for 5 minutes.
• Turn the dough on to a well-floured board and form into two balls. Roll each ball into a circle and cut into eight wedge-shaped pieces. Roll each wedge out to a nice firm, thin shape.
• Place on a very lightly greased baking sheet and bake in the oven for 8–10 minutes, or until lightly golden at the edges. Cool the oatcakes on a wire rack and store them in an airtight container.

Note: This recipe is based on one by the wartime nutritionist and cook, Doris Grant.

★ 1¼ cups/150g old-fashioned oats ground to a coarse meal in a coffee grinder
1 tsp unsalted butter
a pinch of sea salt
½ cup/125g boiling water

moist apple bread

Makes 1 2lb/1kg loaf

- Preheat the oven to 350°F/180°C. Lightly grease and line a 2lb/1kg loaf pan.
- Mix together the flour, sugar, baking powder, and spices in a large mixing bowl. In a separate bowl, mix together the butter, tea, and beaten egg. Beat the mixture into the dry ingredients, stirring until smooth. Fold in the apples, golden raisins and nuts.
- Pour into the prepared pan and bake in the oven for 1 hour, or until the cake is well-risen and indicates it is dry in the middle when tested with a skewer.

★ 1½ cups/180g whole wheat flour
½ cup/125g brown sugar
1 tsp baking powder
★ 1 tsp cinnamon
★ ½ tsp ground cloves
★ ¼ tsp grated nutmeg
★ 8 tbsp/125g butter, melted
⅔ cup/150ml cold tea
★ 1 egg, beaten
★ 6oz/180g apples, unpeeled and grated
★ 2½oz/75g golden raisins
★ ⅓ cup/75g walnuts or pecans, roughly chopped

apricot scones

Makes 16

- Preheat the oven to 350°F/180°C. Lightly grease a baking sheet, or cover it with a piece of baking parchment cut to size.
- Sift the flour, soda, salt, and baking powder into a mixing bowl, returning the bran left in the sifter to the bowl. Rub in the butter with your fingertips and mix in the sugar. (Alternatively, process the flour, baking powder, butter, and sugar together in a food processor.) Add the apricots, golden raisins, and sunflower seeds and stir in. Mix in enough milk and water to bind the mixture without making it wet.
- Divide the dough in half and roll each half into a circle on a lightly floured surface to a thickness of about 1¾in/4cm. Cut the dough circles into eight triangular sections.
- Place the trianges on the prepared baking sheet and bake in the oven for about 15 minutes until golden on top. Serve the scones warm, split and buttered. Leftovers can be toasted.

★ 4 cups/500g whole wheat flour
½ tsp soda
¼ tsp salt
2 tsp baking powder
★ 6 tbsp/90g butter, diced
⅓ cup/60g dark brown sugar
★ 4oz/125g ready-to-eat dried apricots, washed, dried and cut into raisin-size pieces
★ 2oz/60g golden raisins
★ 2oz/60g sunflower seeds
★ 1¼ cups/300ml milk and water mixed

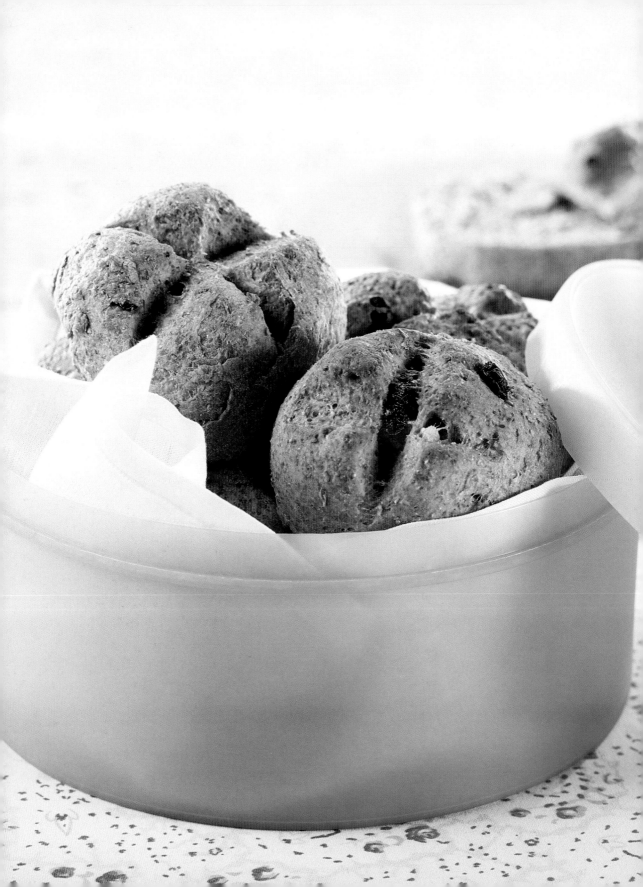

hot cross buns

Makes 12

These buns are delicious for breakfast. Try them split and toasted.

• Mix 1 cup/125g of the flour with the sugar. Sprinkle the mixture over the yeast in a mixing bowl and stir in the milk and water. Leave the mixture in a warm place for 20–30 minutes until it is frothy.

• Meanwhile, mix the remaining flour with the allspice and salt. Add the brown sugar, currants, and mixed peel. Stir the melted butter and beaten egg into the frothy yeast mixture. Gradually fold in the flour mixture and mix to a smooth dough.

• Knead the dough on a lightly floured surface until it is smooth and elastic. Divide the dough into 12 pieces and shape them into flattish round little buns. Make two slashes to form a cross on top of each one. Set the buns well apart on a greased and floured baking sheet and let them rise again in a warm place for about 30 minutes, or until they have doubled in size.

• While the dough is rising, preheat the oven to 375°F/190°C. Bake the buns in the oven for 15–20 minutes until golden on top.

Illustrated left

★ 4 cups/500g whole wheat flour
1 tsp sugar
1 tbsp active dried yeast
★ ⅔ cup/150ml lukewarm milk
★ ¼ cup/60ml hand-hot water
1 tsp allspice
1 tsp fine salt
½ cup/60g light brown sugar
★ 1oz/30g currants
1oz/30g mixed peel
★ 4 tbsp/60g butter, melted
★ 1 egg, beaten

green tea bread

Makes 1 2lb/1kg loaf

• Put the dried fruit in a large bowl and stir in the tea and sugar. Cover and set aside to soak overnight.

• Next day, preheat the oven to 350°F/180°C. Lightly grease a 2lb/1kg loaf pan.

• Add the remaining ingredients to the dried-fruit mixture and beat well. Pour the mixture into the prepared loaf pan, pushing the mixture into the corners of the pan.

• Transfer to the preheated oven and bake for 1 hour 15 minutes, or until a skewer inserted into the center of the bread comes out clean. Turn the bread out of the pan and let it cool on a wire rack.

★ 12oz/375g seedless raisins and raisins, mixed
1½ cups/300ml green tea (or your favorite tea)
1 cup/180g soft brown sugar
★ 2 cups/250g whole wheat flour
½ tsp baking powder
¼ tsp salt
★ 1 egg
1 tsp mixed spice
★ grated zest of 1 lemon
★ 3oz/90g mixed chopped almonds, walnuts, and hazelnuts

★ = superfood

blueberry muffins

Makes 12

• Preheat the oven to 350°F/180°C. Put 12 paper muffin cases into a muffin pan.
• Sift the flours, baking powder and mixed spice into a mixing bowl, putting the bran in the strainer back into the bowl. Beat together the milk, butter, egg, lemon juice, and sugar in a bowl. Make a well in the center of the flour mixture and pour in half the milk mixture. Gently fold it in, then add the rest and stir it in. Fold in the blueberries.
• Spoon the mixture into the muffin cups. Bake in the oven for about 20 minutes, until well-risen and golden on top. Take the muffins out of the pan and let them cool on a wire rack.

¾ cup/100g self-rising flour
★ ½ cup/60g whole wheat flour
1 tsp baking powder
½ tsp cinnamon
★ ½ cup/125ml milk
★ ½ cup/60g butter, melted
★ 1 large egg
★ 2 tsp lemon juice
½ cup/90g soft brown sugar
★ ¾ cup/90g fresh blueberries

shortbread trees

Makes 12

• Preheat the oven to 300°F/150°C. Put the butter, sugar, flour, and rice flour or cornstarch in a mixing bowl and rub together with your fingertips. Then work the mixture together with your hands into a smooth dough.
• Put the dough on a work surface lightly dusted with confectioners sugar and roll out to a thickness of about ½in/1cm. Cut out 12 "trees" – tall triangles with tree trunks are easy shapes. Press the nuts vertically into the tree shapes to achieve a spiky effect.
• Place the trees on a baking sheet and bake for 30 minutes. Cool them on a wire rack and, when completely cold, store in an airtight pan.

★ 8 tbsp/125g butter, softened
¼ cup/60g golden sugar
★ 1 cup/125g whole wheat flour
★ ½ cup/60g rice flour or cornstarch
★ ½ cup/60g pine nuts or slivered almonds

carrot cake

Makes 1 8in (20cm) cake

• Preheat the oven to 350°F/180°C. Grease and line an 8in/20cm cake pan.
• Beat the eggs and sugar together to a creamy mix. Add the remaining ingredients and mix to a batter. Spoon into the prepared pan.
• Bake in the preheated oven for 20–25 minutes, until well-risen and nicely brown on top. A skewer inserted into the middle of the cake should come out clean when it is completely baked.

★ 2 eggs
⅛ cup/100g brown sugar
★ 6oz/180g carrots, grated
★ ⅓ cup/90ml light vegetable oil
★ 1cup/100g whole wheat flour
½ tsp soda
★ 1 tsp ground cinnamon
★ ½ tsp ground nutmeg
★ ⅓ cup/60g raisins
★ ½ cup/60g chopped walnuts

banana & walnut bread

**Makes 1
1kg (2lb) loaf**

• Preheat the oven to 350°F/180°C. Line a 2lb/1kg loaf pan with greased waxed paper or baking parchment.

• Cream the cottage cheese and sugar together until well blended. Gradually beat in the eggs. Add the nuts and bananas and mix well. Add the flour, soda, and salt, mixing them in well. Spoon the mixture into the prepared pan, pressing it into the corners.

• Bake in the oven for 40–45 minutes, or until a skewer inserted into the center of the bread comes out clean. Cool on a wire rack and serve sliced and lightly buttered.

★ **1 cup/250g cottage cheese, pressed through a strainer**
½ **cup/125g brown sugar**
★ **3 eggs, beaten**
★ ½ **cup/60g chopped walnuts**
★ **2 bananas, mashed**
★ **2 cups/250g whole wheat flour**
1½ **tsp soda**
½ **tsp salt**

banana & almond muffins

Makes 12

• Heat the oven to 400°F/200°C. Lightly grease a 12-cup muffin pan.

• Put the flour, baking powder, baking soda, and salt in a large mixing bowl and mix well together. Mix the eggs, bananas, sugar, oil, buttermilk, and vanilla extract in a separate bowl and then pour them into the dry ingredients. Mix them together until just combined. (Be careful not to overmix or the muffins will be tough.) Fold in the almonds. Fill each muffin cup to the rim with batter.

• Bake for 25–30 minutes, until firm to the touch and golden on top. Cool the muffins for 2–3 minutes and serve them warm or at room temperature.

1½ **cups/180g all-purpose flour**
1½ **tsp baking powder**
1½ **tsp baking soda**
½ **tsp salt**
★ **2 eggs**
★ **6 large ripe bananas, thoroughly mashed**
1 **cup/250g dark brown sugar**
★ ⅓ **cup/90ml sunflower oil**
★ ⅓ **cup/90ml buttermilk**
½ **tsp vanilla extract**
★ **1 cup/100g almonds, toasted and chopped**

satisfying suppers

The last meal of the day is a great opportunity for you and your children to quickly and easily prepare a nutrition-packed meal together and eat with one another in a **relaxed atmosphere.**

haddock moussaka

★ = superfood

Serves 2

• Preheat the oven to 375°F/190°C. Lightly butter a shallow ovenproof dish.
• Slice the fish into very small pieces, checking very carefully for the tiniest bones and removing them. Put the fish in a dish and sprinkle with the lemon juice. Cook the zucchini for just a minute in boiling water then drain, pat dry, and put it on top of the fish. Beat the egg and milk together, add the nutmeg and dill, and pour over the fish and zucchini. Sprinkle the wheatgerm on top.
• Put the dish in a small roasting pan and pour in cold water to come halfway up the side of the dish. Bake in the oven for 45 minutes, until the top is golden brown.

★ butter, for greasing
★ 6oz/180g haddock fillets
★ 1 tsp lemon juice
2 small zucchini, thinly sliced
★ 1 egg
★ ⅔ cup/150ml warm milk
★ pinch of nutmeg
a little fresh dill
★ 1 tbsp wheatgerm

zoë's shrimp & vegetable stir-fry

Illustrated right

Serves 4

Teenager Zoë has been an enthusiastic cook since she was nine. This is one of her favorite recipes.
• Heat the oil in a frying pan. Add the shrimp and garlic, stir-fry for 2 minutes, then remove with a slotted spoon and set aside. Put the pepper, carrot, green beans, and corn in the pan and stir-fry for 2–3 minutes. Pour the stock into the pan, bring to a boil, lower the heat, and simmer for about 10 minutes, until the vegetables are tender.
• Meanwhile, cook the noodles according to the package directions and drain. Return the garlic and shrimp to the pan, add the noodles, and stir in the chili and soy sauces.

★ 3 tbsp olive oil
★ 8oz/250g cooked shrimp, thawed if frozen, drained and blotted dry
★ 1 clove garlic, chopped
★ 1 red bell pepper, seeded and chopped
★ 1 large carrot, finely diced
★ a handful of green beans, chopped
★ ¾ cup/125g corn kernels
4½ cups/550ml vegetable stock
7oz/200g egg noodles
1 tsp sweet chili sauce
dash of soy sauce

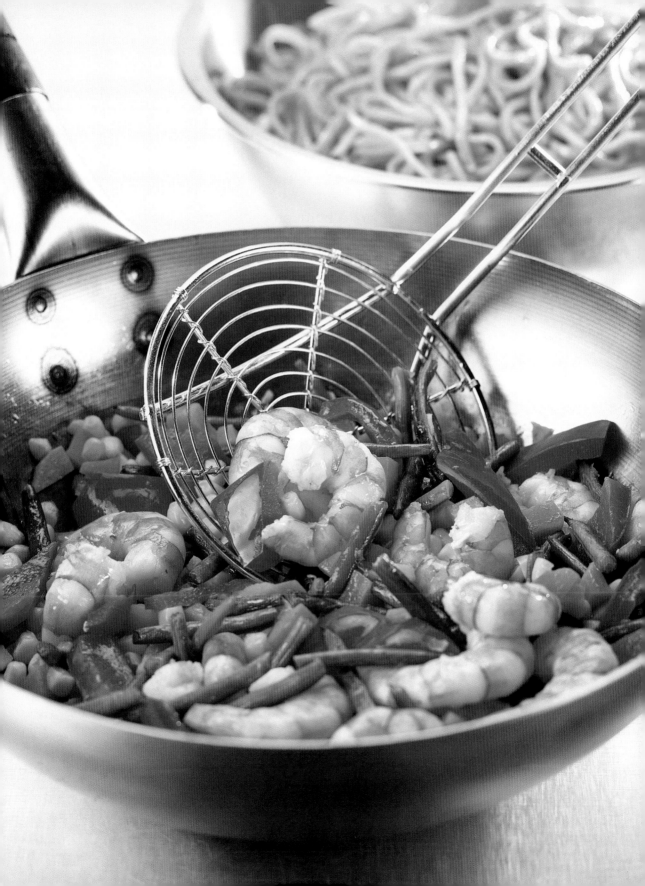

poached chicken

Serves 4

A baby can join in this family meal if you purée a little chicken breast meat with some of the vegetables.
• Put the butter and oil in a heavy-bottomed saucepan or flameproof casserole and heat until the butter is melted. Put the chicken in the pan and brown it on all sides. Add the water or stock, leeks, onion, carrots, and bouquet garni and bring to a boil.
• Reduce the heat, cover the pan, and simmer gently for 45–60 minutes, until the chicken is cooked through and tender. Add the potatoes after 25 minutes' cooking time.

★ = superfood

★ 1 tsp of butter
★ 1 tbsp olive oil
★ 1 medium-sized chicken
1¼ cups/300ml water or vegetable stock
★ white part of 2 leeks
★ 1 large onion, chopped
★ 2 carrots, sliced
★ bouquet garni (sprig of thyme, a bayleaf and a sprig of parsley)
★ 2 large potatoes, peeled and cut into chunks

rabbit with prunes

Serves 4

This is a popular Tuscan dish in which sweet, juicy prunes are a nice match with rabbit, which is sometimes on the dry side. Young children may prefer the dish made with chicken.
• Heat the oil in an ovenproof casserole. Add the onions and fry over a medium heat until soft. Remove from the casserole with a slotted spoon. Roll the rabbit pieces in the flour, put them in the casserole, and brown in the hot oil, adding a little more oil, if necessary.
• When the rabbit pieces are browned all over, add the onions, wine, prunes, thyme, bay leaf, and seasoning. Bring to a boil, cover the pan, reduce the heat, and simmer for about an hour, or until the rabbit is cooked through and is tender.

★ 2 tbsp olive oil
★ 2 onions, chopped
★ 1 rabbit, chopped into 8 pieces
★ 1 tbsp whole wheat flour
⅔ cup/150ml red wine
★ 12 prunes, well washed
★ few sprigs of thyme
1 bay leaf
salt and black pepper

real fish sticks

Serves 1

• Cut the fish into strips, feeling carefully for any bones which may have been left after filleting. Dip the fish strips first in the matzo meal, then in the egg. Heat the vegetable oil in a frying pan, add the fish and shallow-fry for 2–3 minutes on each side.

★ 4oz/125g white fish fillets
2–3 tbsp matzo meal
★ 1 egg, beaten
vegetable oil, for frying

roast chicken puréed with vegetables

Makes 1–2 portions

6-9 months

This highly nutritious baby meal is best made with all organic foods. Make sure the roast chicken is completely cooked through: when pierced with a skewer the juices from the thickest part of the thigh must run clear, not pink. The peas and corn can be either fresh or frozen, but not canned.

• Cut off any skin from the piece of chicken breast and chop the meat finely. Set aside. Cook the pumpkin, peas, and corn in unsalted water until soft. Drain the vegetables, keeping some of the vegetable water in case you need to thin the purée a little. Purée the chicken meat and vegetables together in a food mill, using the coarse disk.

★ small piece skinless breast meat from a roasted chicken
★ 2oz/60g fresh pumpkin, cubed
1 tbsp peas, fresh or frozen
★ 1 tbsp corn kernels, fresh or frozen

rosti-topped fish pie

Serves 4

• Preheat the oven to 400°F/200°C. Put the fish in a saucepan and pour in the milk. Bring to a simmer and cover the pan. Turn off the heat and let it stand for 10 minutes. The fish will be just cooked but still succulent.

• Meanwhile, peel the par-boiled potatoes and coarsely grate them. Strain the milk from the fish into a measuring cup. Flake the fish, discarding all skin and the bones.

• Melt 2tbsp/30g of the butter in a small saucepan and stir in the flour. Gradually stir in the milk from the fish over a low heat, so that the sauce thickens slowly. Simmer the sauce, stirring, until it is smooth.

• Stir the flaked fish, chopped eggs, and parsley into the sauce. Season with pepper and a little salt. Add a little grated nutmeg. Spoon the mixture into an ovenproof dish.

• Melt the remaining butter, toss the grated potatoes in it and spoon them on top of the pie. Bake in the oven for 15–20 minutes until the potatoes are crisp and golden on the top.

★ 8oz/250g white fish
★ 8oz/250g natural smoked fish
★ 2½ cups/600ml milk
★ 1lb/500g waxy potatoes, par-boiled in their skins
★ 4 tbsp/60g butter
¼ cup/30g all-purpose flour
★ 2 hard-boiled eggs, peeled and chopped
★ 2 tbsp chopped fresh parsley
sea salt and freshly ground black pepper
★ nutmeg

irish stew

Serves 2

There should be plenty of delicious stew here to serve a hungry grown-up and a toddler.
- Trim as much excess fat as possible off the lamb. Put the meat in a small flameproof casserole or a heavy-bottomed saucepan. Cover it with the onions and top with the potato slices. Add the thyme and pour in the vegetable stock.
- Bring to a boil, reduce the heat to very low, cover the pan, and cook for at least 1½ hours. By this time the potatoes and onions should have melted into a delicious savory purée, and the lamb should be very tender.
- Pick the meat off the bones (if using lamb chops) and mash it into the vegetables.

- ★ 3 lamb chops or 12oz/375g stewing lamb
- ★ 2 small onions, thinly sliced
- ★ 2 potatoes, thickly sliced
- ★ sprig of fresh thyme
- 5 tbsp vegetable stock

black bean chili

Serves 6

Omitting the lamb from this recipe turns it into a vegetarian dish.
- Heat some olive oil in a large, heavy-bottomed saucepan or flameproof casserole. Add the carrots, celery, and garlic and stir-fry until the vegetables begin to turn golden. Add the chilies, ground cumin, and ground coriander. Fry for a few more minutes. Add the minced lamb and stir-fry until the meat is browned all over.
- Pour the tomatoes and drained beans into the pan and season well. Cover the pan and simmer for about 45 minutes, or until the beans are melting and tender. Check the pan occasionally and stir the contents. If the mixture seems to be getting dry, add a little stock or water to moisten it. Add seasoning to taste and the cilantro towards the end of the cooking time, to preserve its color and flavor.
- Serve the chili in bowls with a dollop of sour cream, some guacamole, and lots of warm tortillas or corn bread to soak up the juices.

- olive oil, for frying
- ★ 2 carrots, very finely diced
- ★ 2 sticks celery, very finely diced
- ★ 6 cloves garlic, finely chopped
- ★ 1–2 red chilies, finely chopped
- ★ 2 tsp ground cumin
- ★ 2 tsp ground coriander
- ★ 1lb/500g lean ground lamb
- ★ 1lb 10oz/800g canned plum tomatoes
- ★ 1lb/500g black beans, soaked overnight in plenty of cold water, and drained
- sea salt and black pepper
- ★ bunch of cilantro, chopped
- sour cream, guacamole, and tortillas or corn bread, to serve

herbed kofta kebabs

Serves 4

Soak eight wooden skewers or satay sticks in water for an hour before making these kebabs.

• Put the lamb in a large bowl and mix in the spices and herbs. Season well with salt and pepper. Heat the olive oil in a frying pan. Add the onion and garlic and fry until soft. Stir into the lamb mixture and mix everything together well.

• Take a little of the lamb mixture and shape it into an oval in your hands. Thread the oval onto a wooden skewer and continue with the process until all the lamb mixture is used up. Cook the kebabs under a hot broiler for 5 minutes on each side, or char-broil or barbecue them.

• Serve with natural yogurt with a little freshly chopped mint added. Couscous or bulgur wheat salad would go very well with the kebabs.

★ 8oz/250g lean groundlamb
★ 1 tsp ground coriander
★ 1 tsp ground cumin
★ 2 tsp chopped fresh mint, plus extra to serve
★ 2 tsp chopped fresh cilantro
★ 2 tsp chopped fresh parsley
sea salt and black pepper
★ 1 tbsp olive oil
★ 1 red onion, finely chopped
★ 1 clove garlic, minced
natural yogurt, to serve

south of france omelette

Serves 4

For the more adventurous breakfast eaters, this is a very satisfying and tasty omelette that children enjoy for any meal, perhaps accompanied by of a few little potatoes roasted in their skins. You can be experimental with the vegetables – it would be a very good way of using up a few spoonfuls of leftover ratatouille or some roasted vegetables.

• Heat 1 tablespoon of the oil in a frying pan. Add the tomatoes, eggplant, and garlic and fry them until they are cooked through and almost a purée.

• Break the eggs into a bowl and add the fresh herbs and seasoning. Beat the eggs with a fork until just blended and stir in half the vegetable mixture.

• Heat the remaining olive oil in a frying pan. Pour the egg mixture evenly into the pan. Cook until the underside is firm and golden brown; the omelette is now ready to lift and fold over. Spoon the rest of the vegetable mixture into the middle of the folded-over omelette. Slide the omelette on to a warm plate and serve immediately.

★ 2 tbsp olive oil
★ 2 ripe tomatoes, diced
★ 1 small eggplant, diced
★ 2 cloves garlic, finely chopped
★ 8 eggs
★ 2 tsp chopped fresh parsley
★ 2 tsp chopped fresh chives
2 tsp chopped fresh chervil
salt and pepper

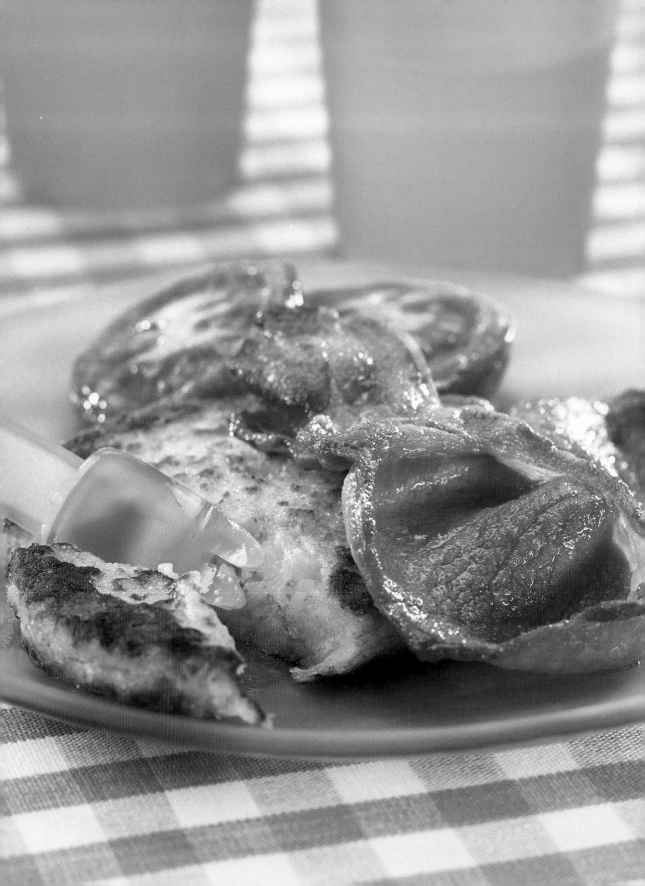

cauliflower & broccoli cheese

★ = superfood

Serves 4

• Preheat the oven to 350°F/180°C. Butter a gratin dish thoroughly.

• Put the cauliflower and broccoli florets in a saucepan, add the milk, and cook until just tender. Drain the vegetables, reserving the milk, and put them in the gratin dish.

• Melt the butter in a small non-stick saucepan. Stir in the flour, 1 tablespoon of the cheese, the mustard, and seasoning to taste. Stir in the hot milk, a little at a time, until you have a smooth creamy sauce.

• Heat through and pour over the cauliflower and broccoli. Scatter the remaining cheese on top and bake in the oven for 15–20 minutes. For a nice browned surface, finish the dish under a hot broiler.

★ 1 small cauliflower, broken into small florets

★ 1 small head of broccoli, broken into small florets

★ 2 cups/500ml milk

★ 4 tbsp/60g butter

★ 1 tbsp whole wheat flour

★ ½ cup/60g grated hard cheese, such as mature Cheddar

1 tsp Dijon mustard

salt and black pepper

potato cakes with broiled bacon

Serves 4

This is an excellent way to use up boiled or mashed potatoes without going to extra trouble. The dough should be squeezed from hand to hand until it looks smooth and unbreakable.

• Mash the warm potatoes thoroughly with the butter, salt, and pepper. Work in the flour. Taking about 2 tablespoons of the mixture at a time, make eight potato cakes, using some extra flour on the surface and squeezing and patting the dough into flat rounds that are nice and smooth in texture.

• Heat a little olive oil in a frying pan, add the potato cakes and fry them until crisp and golden on each side. While the potato cakes are cooking, broil the bacon and drain it on paper towels.

Illustrated left

• Serve the potato cakes with the bacon and with broiled tomato halves, if your children like them.

★ 1lb/500g cooked potatoes

★ 1 tbsp of butter

salt and pepper

★ 2 tbsp whole wheat flour, plus extra for coating

★ olive oil, for frying

★ 8 strips bacon

★ broiled tomato halves, to serve (optional)

vegetable couscous

★ = superfood

Serves 2

If a child insists on having meat with this, fry a few small pieces of chicken with the onion.

- Heat a little olive oil in a frying pan. Add the onion and fry until golden. Add the carrots, zucchini, red bell pepper, and ground cumin and continue to fry for a few minutes.
- Add the tomatoes, a little salt, and the cilantro. Simmer for about 10 minutes, or until the vegetables are cooked and nicely tender. Add the chickpeas and heat through.
- While the vegetables are cooking, steam the couscous, according to package directions. Serve the vegetables and steamed couscous together.

★ olive oil, for frying
★ 1 onion, finely chopped
★ 2 carrots, halved lengthwise and sliced
1 small zucchini, halved lengthwise and sliced
★ ½ red bell pepper, seeded and chopped
★ 1 tsp (or more to taste) ground cumin
★ 2 tomatoes, skinned and diced
salt
★ 1–2 tbsp cilantro
★ 13oz/400g canned chickpeas, drained
★ ¼ cup/150g couscous

vegetable samosas

Makes approx. 16

- Boil the potato cubes in lightly salted water for about 10 minutes, or until soft. Drain well. In a separate pan bring enough water to a boil to just cover the chopped vegetables and cook them until tender but still crisp. Drain well.
- Put the vegetables and potatoes into a bowl. Add the curry powder or paste, cheese, and salt and pepper. Mix everything well. Preheat the oven to 375°F/190°C.
- Melt the olive oil and butter in a small saucepan. Lay out one sheet of filo pastry and brush it with the melted butter and oil. Place another sheet on top and brush again. Now cut the pastry lengthwise into strips about 3in/7cm wide. Put a heaping teaspoonful of filling at one end of a strip. Fold the pastry diagonally across so that it makes a triangle. Keep folding over along the length of the strip until your triangle is completed. Brush the outside with butter and roll the samosa in poppy or black sesame seeds. Repeat with all your pastry and filling. You should get about 16.
- Put the samosas on a baking sheet and bake in the oven for 15–20 minutes, until golden. Serve the samosas while they are still warm.

2 potatoes, cut into ½ inch cubes
★ 4oz/125g finely chopped vegetables – use combinations of favorite vegetables, such as carrots, beans, peas, spinach, corn, cauliflower, and parsnips
1 tsp mild curry powder or paste
★ 2 tbsp cream cheese or cottage cheese
salt and black pepper
★ 1 tbsp olive oil
★ 2 tbsp/30g butter, melted
8 sheets filo pastry
★ poppy seeds or black sesame seeds

brown rice four ways

Brown rice is sustaining comfort food for a simple meal. Once cooked, it can be served in many ways, not just the four suggested below.

• Preheat the oven to 325°F/160°C. Wash the rice thoroughly in several changes of water, then drain well. Put it in an ovenproof casserole and cover with water to about ½ inch above the surface of the rice. Cover tightly with a lid, put in the oven and bake for about 40 minutes. If the rice is still a little soggy after this time, put it back in the oven for a few minutes without the lid.

To make a delicious meal of the cooked rice, try the following ideas – or adapt them to your own and your children's liking:

• Serve with a teaspoon of butter, some grated cheese, and a little chopped fresh mint stirred into it.

• Serve it with Roasted Vegetables (see page 174).

• Make it into a salad. Add a couple of tablespoons of extra-virgin olive oil, a teaspoon of lemon juice, a pinch of sea salt, freshly ground black pepper, a finely chopped garlic clove, and any of the following: in summer, chopped ripe red tomatoes, cucumber, scallions, avocado, and fresh basil; in winter, small chunks of celery, fennel, raisins, sunflower seeds, or pine nuts tossed in a little oil and with chopped fresh parsley, or cilantro sprinkled on top.

• Serve it with apple purée and a little cinnamon. A classic French food for anyone who has been unwell or suffered a digestive upset, this is also a perfect meal-in-itself supper.

★ 1¼ cup/250g brown rice

water (see method)

roasted vegetables

★ = superfood

Serves 4

Served these vegetables with plain brown rice (see page 173), couscous, or bulgur for an appetizing and colorful supper. The vegetables are also a delicious accompaniment to the Sunday roast, broiled fish or meat, or to a simple omelette.

• Preheat the oven to 400°F/200°C. Arrange all the vegetables and garlic in a shallow roasting pan. Add the olive oil and push all the vegetables around until they are well-coated with the oil. Sprinkle with a little salt and pepper.

• Roast in the oven for about 40 minutes, giving them a stir once or twice. They should be tender, and just starting to turn golden-brown. Serve sprinkled with the chopped fresh herbs.

★ 1 red bell pepper, cored, seeded, and cut into chunks
★ 1 yellow bell pepper, cored, seeded, and cut into chunks
★ 2 onions, quartered
2 medium or 4 small zucchini, thickly sliced
★ 8 cherry tomatoes
★ 4 cloves garlic
★ 4 tbsp olive oil
salt and black pepper
★ bunch of cilantro, basil, or parsley

bubble & squeak

Serves 4

Traditionally, this is made with leftover cooked cabbage and potatoes, but you can use up Brussels sprouts, peas, and broccoli this way too. The one cardinal rule is that there should be more potatoes than greens.

• Break up the cooked potatoes with a fork, add a little milk and the butter and roughly mash. Add the shredded cooked greens to the potato and mix together. Shape the mixture into one big cake or four smaller patties and dust with seasoned flour.

• Heat the olive oil in a frying pan. Add the cakes of bubble and squeak, press down firmly, and fry on both sides till golden brown.

★ 1lb/500g cooked potatoes
★ milk, for mashing
★ 1 tsp butter
★ 10oz/300g shredded and cooked cabbage
seasoned flour, for dusting
★ 2–3 tbsp olive oil

broccoli & anchovy pasta

Serves 4

• Bring a large saucepan of lightly salted boiling water, to which you have added a dash of vegetable oil, to a boil. Add the broccoli florets and cook until barely tender. Drain, reserving the cooking water.

• Add more water to the broccoli cooking water, if necessary, since pasta needs to cook in plenty of water. Bring the water back to a boil, add the pasta and cook it until it is tender but still a little firm – or "al dente," as the Italians describe it.

• While the pasta is cooking, heat the oil in a frying pan. Add the garlic and fry until just translucent. Add the anchovies or anchovy paste and the broccoli florets, stir all together in the oil, and add freshly ground black pepper. Keep hot until the pasta is cooked. Drain the pasta, return it to its pan, add the broccoli sauce, and toss well. Stir in the cheese and serve piping hot.

★ 1 medium head broccoli, broken into small florets
★ 12oz/375g pasta shapes, such as orecchiette, spaghettini or conchigli
★ 5 tbsp olive oil
★ 2 cloves garlic, finely chopped
★ 3–4 anchovy fillets, finely chopped or 1 squeeze of anchovy paste
black pepper
★ 3 tbsp freshly grated Parmesan cheese

pasta with avocado sauce

Serves 4

In this delectable simple pasta dish the taste depends on the freshness and quality of the ingredients. With its creamy delicate texture, this is a pasta which even young children will enjoy.

• Scoop out the flesh of the two avocados – which should be perfectly ripe, deep yellow and unblemished – into the bowl in which you will serve the pasta. Mash the avocado flesh well. Add the lemon juice and mash again. Add the crushed garlic and stir it in. Add the seasoning to taste, followed by the olive oil, and mash thoroughly to make a creamy sauce.

• Cook the pasta in plenty of boiling water. Test to see if it is nearly done, add a tablespoon or so of the pasta cooking water to the sauce, and mix in thoroughly. When the pasta is cooked – it should be tender, but still slightly firm – drain it well. Tip it on top of the sauce and toss very thoroughly to combine before serving.

Note: you can use more or less lemon juice, garlic or olive oil according to family taste.

★ 2 ripe avocados
★ juice of 1 lemon
★ 1 fat garlic clove, crushed
salt and black pepper
★ 1 tbsp olive oil
★ 12oz/375g dried pasta, preferably tagliatelle

pasta sauces

★ = superfood

Pasta is wholesome fast food that the right sauces can turn into delicious and healthy feasts. On these pages you will find some great, easy-to-prepare sauces that work well with all the huge variety of pasta shapes, fresh or dried, available today. When cooking pasta for a main meal, allow approximately 1lb/500g to serve four.

raw tomato sauce

Serves 4

- Put the tomato quarters in a food processor with the basil, parsley, garlic, and seasoning and process into a thick sauce. Put the sauce in the dish in which you will serve the pasta.
- Cook your chosen pasta until it is al dente (see page 175). Drain it well and tip it out onto the sauce. Stir together very quickly and sprinkle the grated Parmesan cheese on top, if using. Serve immediately.

★ **12oz/375g ripe fresh tomatoes, skinned and quartered**
★ **8–10 basil leaves**
★ **handful of fresh parsley**
★ **2 garlic cloves, lightly crushed**
salt and black pepper
★ **freshly grated Parmesan cheese (optional)**

raw tomato & red bell pepper sauce

Serves 4

- Put the tomato quarters in a food processor with the pepper(s), parsley, grated Parmesan cheese, and 2–3 tablespoons of the olive oil. Process to a thick sauce, adding more olive oil through the top of the processor as needed.
- Cook your chosen pasta (see page 175) and drain well. Add the sauce and stir it through. Serve at once.

★ **5oz/150g ripe fresh tomatoes, skinned and quartered**
★ **1 large red bell pepper, or 1 small red and 1 small yellow bell pepper, cored, seeded, and quartered**
★ **1 tbsp fresh parsley**
★ **2 tbsp freshly grated Parmesan cheese**
★ **4–5 tbsp olive oil**

mozzarella, tomato & parmesan sauce

Serves 4

- A couple of hours before you plan to eat, peel and finely chop the tomatoes. Put them in a bowl with the olive oil, basil leaves, oregano, and grated Parmesan. Leave to macerate for 2 hours.
- Put the cubes of mozzarella into the dish in which you plan to serve the pasta.
- Cook your chosen pasta until it is al dente (see page 175). Drain it well and tip it on top of the mozzarella cubes, stirring very quickly so that the melting cheese disperses throughout the pasta.
- Add the tomato mixture, stir again, and serve.

★ **12oz/375g ripe fresh tomatoes**
★ **6 tbsp olive oil**
★ **handful of fresh basil leaves, roughly torn**
★ **sprig of fresh oregano**
★ **3 tbsp freshly grated Parmesan cheese**
★ **5oz/150g mozzarella cheese, cubed**

tomato & anchovy sauce

Serves 4

Older children will enjoy this Italian classic. Add just a touch of anchovy – perhaps a small squeeze of anchovy paste from a tube - the first time you make this sauce. It can be made in advance and reheated to serve with your chosen pasta.

• Heat the oil in a small saucepan, add the garlic and cook gently for 2–3 minutes. Add the tomatoes, olives, and oregano. Simmer very gently for a few minutes then add the chopped anchovies. Cook a few minutes longer until the anchovies have softened and blended with the sauce.

• Add the parsley and a twist or two of pepper. The anchovies will give the sauce all the salt it needs.

★ ½ cup/100ml olive oil
★ 3 cloves garlic, finely chopped
★ 7oz/200g canned chopped tomatoes
2oz/60g pitted black olives, chopped
pinch of dried oregano
3–4 anchovy fillets, well rinsed, dried, and finely chopped
★ 2 tbsp finely chopped fresh parsley
black pepper

ham & mushroom sauce

Serves 4

• Melt the butter in a small saucepan, add the onion and garlic, and cook until softened. Add the mushrooms and let them color a little. Add the ham and fry gently until it has taken on a little color. Add the wine, nutmeg, and seasoning.

• Simmer over a very low heat for 5–10 minutes, adding a little boiling water if the sauce gets too dry.

• Cook the pasta until it is al dente (see page 175), drain well, and stir in the sauce. Serve immediately.

★ 4 tbsp/60g butter
★ 1 onion, finely chopped
★ 1 clove garlic, finely chopped
3oz/90g fresh mushrooms, finely sliced
★ 4oz/125g cooked ham, cubed
½ cup/125ml white wine
★ pinch of grated nutmeg
salt and black pepper

classic bolognese sauce

Serves 4

• Melt the butter with the oil in a saucepan. Add the vegetables and soften them in the fat. Add the ground beef and fry gently until the meat begins to brown. Add the wine and cook until most of it has been absorbed. Add the tomatoes and herbs, turn the heat up, and boil for a couple of minutes.

• Turn the heat down and simmer gently for about an hour, adding a little stock from time to time if the sauce looks too dry: it should be dense but liquid.

• Traditionally, this sauce is eaten with tagliatelle. Cook the pasta (see page 175) and drain it well. Stir in the sauce. Serve with the grated Parmesan passed aound separately.

★ 4 tbsp/60g butter
★ 1 tbsp olive oil
★ 1 onion, finely chopped
★ 1 carrot, grated
★ 1 stick celery, finely chopped
★ 7oz/200g lean ground beef
½ cup/125ml red wine
★ 7oz/200g canned chopped tomatoes
★ 1 tbsp chopped fresh parsley
★ sprig of fresh or a pinch of dried thyme
★ 1 bay leaf
a little vegetable stock
salt and black pepper
★ 4 tbsp freshly grated Parmesan cheese

sophie's indonesian vegetable stew

★ = superfood

Serves 2

Four-year-old Sophie van der Zee has been eating spicy savory food like this ever since she graduated from little fruit and vegetable purées: proof that food doesn't have to be bland where babies and toddlers are concerned. The lime leaf gives this dish its lovely special flavor; it can be bought in markets selling Thai or Indonesian foods.

• Heat a little sunflower oil in a frying pan. Add the diced tofu and fry until golden. Drain and set aside. Add a little more oil to the pan, if necessary, and fry the onion and garlic in it until softened. Add the lime leaf, cabbage, pepper, carrots, and beans and fry for 3–4 minutes. Add the coconut milk, salt, to taste, and tofu and let the mixture simmer until the vegetables are tender. Add the corn and heat through. The dish should be soup-like in consistency. Serve it with basmati rice.

★ sunflower oil, for frying
★ 4oz/125g firm tofu, diced
★ 1 onion, chopped
★ 1 clove garlic, chopped
1 lime leaf
★ small wedge white cabbage, chopped
★ ½ red bell pepper, seeded and chopped
★ 2 carrots, sliced
★ 10 butter beans
2–3 cups coconut milk
salt
★ 5oz/150g fresh or frozen corn kernels, drained
basmati rice, to serve

chicken in a wrap

Serves 4

Put all the ingredients, except the flour for coating and the olive oil, into a large bowl. Mix very thoroughly together and set aside for a few minutes to let the flavors mingle. Shape the mixture into four burgers. Toss each burger lightly in the seasoned flour to coat.

• Heat a little olive oil in a frying pan and fry the burgers for 3–4 minutes on each side, until cooked well through. Alternatively, the burgers can be brushed with oil and broiled or baked in a moderately hot oven, turning them once.

• Serve in soft tortillas, with mayonnaise, shreds of crisp lettuce, and slices of avocado. As a variation, put the burgers in warm whole wheat rolls and substitute sour cream for the mayonnaise.

★ 1lb/500g ground chicken
★ 1 tbsp dark soy sauce or tamari sauce
★ 1 tsp grated fresh root ginger
★ 1 clove garlic, crushed
★ 1 tbsp finely chopped cilantro
½ tsp sea salt
black pepper
★ seasoned whole wheat flour, to coat
★ olive oil, for frying
4 soft tortillas, mayonnaise, lettuce and avocado, to serve

Illustrated right

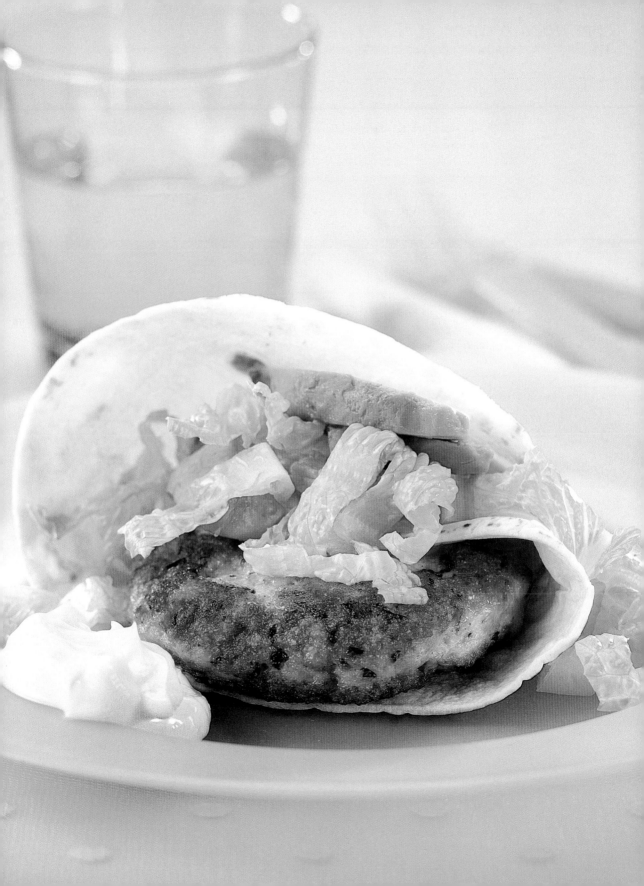

mashed potatoes and celeriac

★ = superfood

Serves 4

Serve this tasty purée with burgers, sausages, roast chicken, or fish dishes.
- Add the lemon juice or vinegar to a large saucepanful of water. Bring the pan to a boil. Slice the knobby skin off the celeriac, cut the celeriac into chunks and drop them into a boiling water.
- Add the potato chunks to the pan. Bring back to a boil, reduce the heat, and simmer for 15–20 minutes, until both vegetables are tender. Drain, reserving the cooking liquid.
- Return the vegetables to the pan and mash them, adding the butter and as much of the reserved liquid as you need to make a creamy purée. (This can be done in a food processor, but be very careful not to over-process or the potatoes will turn to glue.)
- Heat the oil in a small pan. Add the chopped onion and fry very gently until they turn golden, then stir into the purée along with the hot oil from the pan.

★ 1 tbsp lemon juice or white wine vinegar

★ 1 large celeriac

★ 4–5 potatoes, cut into small chunks

★ 1 tsp butter

★ 2 tbsp olive oil

★ 1 small onion, very finely chopped

black pepper

broccoli with spinach

Serves 4

Even people who dislike broccoli may enjoy this spicy, savory way of cooking it taken from Madhur Jaffrey's book *World Vegetarian* (Clarkson Potter). For all but the most grown-up children, leave out the chili and use just a touch of ginger. You could leave out the salt, too. It is delicious cold.
- Bring a large saucepan of water to a boil. Add the spinach and broccoli florets; bring back to a boil and boil rapidly for 3–4 minutes, or until both the spinach and broccoli are tender. Drain into a colander, saving the cooking water for another use. Run cold water over the greens, and let them drain before chopping them finely.
- Heat the oil in a large non-stick frying pan or wok set over a medium-high heat. When hot, put in the onion, garlic, ginger, and chili. Stir-fry until the onion pieces turn brown at the edges. Add the cumin. Stir once, then quickly put the broccoli and spinach into the pan. Stir once or twice and turn the heat to medium. Cook gently, stirring, until the vegetables are just heated through.

★ 12oz/375g spinach, well washed and trimmed

★ 12oz/375g broccoli florets, cut to leave a little of the stems

★ 4 tbsp olive oil

★ 1oz/30g finely chopped onion

★ 1 clove garlic, very finely chopped

★ 2 thin slices fresh ginger, peeled and very finely chopped

★ ½–1 fresh red chili, seeded (optional) and very finely chopped

★ 4 tsp ground cumin

vegetable curry with dal

Serves 4

• First, make the dal. Put the mung beans in a heavy pan, add the water, bring to a boil, reduce the heat, and simmer very gently, skimming off the froth. When the froth has been removed, stir in the turmeric, partly cover the pan, and simmer gently for about 1 hour until the beans are soft. Drain the beans, add salt to taste, and turn the dal into a serving dish. Heat the oil in a small frying pan, add the cumin seeds, and let them sizzle for a couple of minutes. Add the chili and garlic and let them soften but not brown. Tip the mixture into the mung beans and stir well.

• While the dal is cooking, prepare the vegetables. Break broccoli or cauliflower into very small florets, peel and dice potatoes or carrots into small pieces. Blanch in boiling water for 1 minute.

• Heat the oil in a wok or deep frying pan. Add the curry powder, stir for 1 minute, then add the onion and garlic, and stir-fry for 1 more minute. Add the vegetables and stir-fry for 5–10 minutes, until they soften. Add the chickpeas, lemon juice, cilantro, apple, and creamed coconut. Heat for 2–3 minutes. Serve with the dal garnished with cilantro.

★ 1½lbs/750g mixed vegetables, such as broccoli, cauliflower, potatoes, carrots, french beans
★ 3 tbsp peanut oil
2 tsp medium curry powder
★ 1 onion, chopped
★ 3 cloves garlic, chopped
★ 7oz/200g canned chickpeas, drained and rinsed
★ juice of 1 lemon
★ cilantro, chopped
★ 1 eating apple, peeled and chopped
1oz/30g creamed coconut

For the dal:
★ 6oz/180g mung beans, picked over, washed and drained
4½ cups/1 liter water
½ tsp turmeric
a good pinch of salt
2 tbsp vegetable oil
★ 1 tsp cumin seeds
★ chili powder or flakes, to taste
★ 2 cloves garlic
★ cilantro, to garnish

red cabbage with apple & chestnuts

Serves 4

• Cut off the outer leaves of the cabbage and the hard white core. Shred the cabbage finely.

• Make a slit across the round side of each chestnut and put them in a pan of water. Bring to a boil and boil for 10 minutes. Take the chestnuts out of the water one by one and peel and skin them. Break them up roughly and set aside.

• Melt the butter in a large saucepan. Put in the bacon and cabbage. Cover the pan and cook over a medium heat, turning it all over from time to time.

• When the cabbage is beginning to soften, add the apple to the pan, then the vinegar and sugar. Cook the mixture for about 45 minutes, longer if you prefer the cabbage softer. Add the chestnuts at the end, giving them time to warm through. Season to taste before serving.

★ ½ large red cabbage
★ 8oz/250g chestnuts
★ 2 tbsp/30g butter
★ 2 thick slices bacon, chopped
★ 1 large sweet apple, such as Fuji, cored and grated
1–2 tbsp wine vinegar
2–3 tsp brown sugar
salt and black pepper

chickpea veggie burgers

Makes 6 large or 8 medium burgers

• Put the split peas and chickpeas in a food processor and process until very finely chopped, but not reduced to a purée. Heat the oil in a pan, add the chopped onion, and fry gently until soft and golden.

• Put the processed split peas, chickpeas, celery, apple, ground almonds, sunflower seeds, and fried onion in a large bowl. Mix everything well together and season with salt and pepper.

• Shape the mixture into six or eight burgers, pressing them firmly into shape. Dip them first in the beaten egg, then in the breadcrumbs.

• Heat a little sunflower oil in a frying pan and fry the burgers gently for about 7 minutes on each side, until cooked well through. Serve the burgers in whole wheat rolls with watercress or lettuce and a spoonful of mayonnaise.

★ 8oz/250g canned yellow split peas, drained and rinsed
★ 1lb/500g canned chickpeas, drained and rinsed
★ 2 tbsp olive oil
★ 1 large onion, finely chopped
★ 3–4 tender inner sticks celery, finely chopped
★ 1 crisp apple, finely chopped (like Granny Smith)
★ ½ cup/60g ground almonds
★ 1 tbsp sunflower seeds
sea salt and black pepper
★ 1 small egg, beaten
fresh or dried whole wheat breadcrumbs, to coat
★ sunflower oil, for frying
rolls, watercress or lettuce, and mayonnaise, to serve

veggie burgers with spinach cheese topping

Makes 6

• Heat the sunflower oil in a frying pan. Add the onion and fry until soft. Add the garlic and mushrooms. Cook, stirring occasionally, until the juices have evaporated and the vegetables are becoming crisp and golden. Take the pan off the heat and mix in all the remaining ingredients, except the egg, and season to taste. Mix in the beaten egg.

• Shape the mixture into six burgers, pressing each one firmly into a round. Toss them in whole wheat flour to coat. Heat a little vegetable oil in a frying pan and fry the burgers for 3–4 minutes on each side, or until cooked well through. Alternatively, the burgers can be brushed with vegetable oil and broiled or baked in a moderately hot oven.

• Top each cooked burger with a few lightly cooked spinach leaves, and lay a slice of cheese on top of the spinach. Place under a hot broiler until melting and crisp.

• Serve the burgers in whole wheat rolls with added mayonnaise, and a few onion rings.

★ 2 tbsp sunflower oil
★ 1 red onion, finely chopped
★ 2 cloves garlic, crushed
3 cups/250g mushrooms, finely chopped
★ 1 cup/125g almonds, chopped
★ 125g/4oz cooked brown rice or soaked bulgur
★ ⅔ cup/180g carrots, grated
1 tbsp vegetable bouillon
★ handful fresh parsley, chopped
★ 1 tbsp dark soy sauce
sea salt and black pepper
★ 1 egg, beaten
★ whole wheat flour, to coat
★ vegetable oil, for frying

For the topping:
★ lightly cooked spinach leaves
★ slices of cheese
whole wheat rolls and mayonnaise, to serve

nut burgers

Makes 4

• Put the nuts and breadcrumbs in a food processor or blender and process until quite fine.

• Heat the olive oil in a heavy-bottomed saucepan, add the onion and fry gently until soft and golden.

• Off the heat, pour the hot stock into the pan then add the nut mixture, herbs, and seasoning to taste. Mix all the ingredients well together, adding a little more stock if the mixture looks on the dry side.

• Shape the mixture into four burgers and dip them into the whole wheat flour to coat lightly. Heat a little oil in a frying pan and fry the burgers for 3–5 minutes on each side until golden brown.

• Serve the burgers, which are delicious either hot or cold, on whole wheat rolls with a little mayonnaise and shredded lettuce or watercress.

★ 2 cups/250g mixed nuts, such as walnuts, hazelnuts, cashews and peanuts

1 cup/125g whole wheat breadcrumbs

★ 1 tbsp olive oil

★ 1 onion, very finely chopped

1¼ cups/300ml hot vegetable stock, made with vegetable bouillon powder

★ 1 tbsp chopped fresh parsley

★ 2–3 fresh sage leaves, torn in small pieces

sea salt and black pepper

★ whole wheat flour, to coat

★ vegetable oil, for frying

whole wheat rolls, mayonnaise and lettuce or watercress, to serve

rice burgers

Makes 4

• Wash the rice thoroughly and drain it. Bring the bouillon to a boil in a large saucepan. Add the rice, reduce the heat, cover the pan, and cook over a very low heat for about 30 minutes, until all the bouillon is absorbed and the rice is tender.

• While the rice is cooking, put the bread and peanuts in a food processor or blender and process them to crumbs.

• Heat the oil in a large frying pan. Add the onion and fry gently until soft and golden. Reduce the heat and add the parsnip and carrot, stir and fry gently for a few minutes. Add the soy sauce and yeast extract and stir them well in. Add the breadcrumbs and peanut mixture and stir in. Season to taste.

• Tip the fried-onion mixture into a mixing bowl. Add the cooked rice and mix everything well together. Allow the mixture to cool a little, then turn it out on to a floured board. Shape into four fairly thick burgers and chill them in the refrigerator for an hour or so, or overnight.

• Dip the burgers in beaten egg, then coat them with breadcrumbs. Heat a little vegetable oil in a frying pan and fry the burgers for 5–7 minutes on each side until crisp and brown.

★ brown basmati rice, measured up to the 125ml/4fl oz level in a measuring cup

1¼ cups/300ml vegetable bouillon, measured in the same cup as the rice

1 slice whole wheat bread

★ ½ cup/60g dry-roasted peanuts

★ 2 tbsp olive oil

★ 1 onion, finely chopped

1 parsnip (hard core removed), finely grated

★ 1 carrot, finely grated

★ 1 tbsp soy sauce

½ tsp yeast extract

salt and black pepper

★ 1 egg, beaten

dry breadcrumbs, to coat

★ vegetable oil, for frying

bean burgers

★ = superfood

Makes 6

• Heat the oil in a large frying pan. Add the onion and fry over a medium heat until soft and golden. Add the carrots, potato, and mashed beans and continue to cook for about 7 minutes, stirring from time to time, until the vegetables have cooked a little. Add the tomato purée, ketchup, garlic, herbs, soy sauce, and seasoning, and mix well. Mix in the breadcrumbs and mash together to a sticky paste.
• Turn the mixture out on to a floured board and, with floured hands, shape into 6 burgers. Chill in the refrigerator for an hour or two to firm up. Dip the burgers in the beaten egg, then in the breadcrumbs.
• Heat a little olive oil in a frying pan, and fry the burgers over medium heat for about 5 minutes on each side. Serve in whole wheat rolls with chutney, onion rings, and lettuce.

★ **2 tbsp olive oil**
★ **1 large onion, finely chopped**
★ **2 carrots, finely grated**
★ **1 potato, finely grated**
★ **8oz/250g canned red kidney beans, drained, rinsed and mashed**
★ **1 tbsp tomato purée**
★ **1 tbsp tomato ketchup**
★ **1 clove garlic, finely chopped**
pinch of herbs de provence
★ **1 tsp soy sauce**
pinch of salt
black pepper
★ **1 egg, beaten**
1 slice whole wheat bread, crusts removed and crumbed

onion-&-squeak burgers

Makes 6

• Wash and cook the scallions in boiling water until soft. Drain and chop. Mix the eggs, nutmeg, breadcrumbs, mashed potatoes, and seasoning together thoroughly. Mix in the scallions. Shape the mixture into six burgers.
• Heat a little oil in a large frying pan. Add the burgers and fry for 3–5 minutes on each side, until golden brown. Serve with iceberg lettuce, raw onion rings, slices of tomato, and a favorite relish.

★ **12 scallions**
★ **2 eggs, lightly beaten**
★ **good pinch grated nutmeg**
2 slices whole wheat bread, crusts removed, and crumbed
★ **4 cups/375g cold mashed potatoes**
sea salt and black pepper
★ **sunflower oil, for frying**

radar burgers

Makes 4 large or 6 medium burgers

• Heat a little oil in a frying pan. Add the onion and fry gently until soft. Put the beef, carrot, breadcrumbs, and herbs in a bowl. Add the onions and mix well. Shape the mixture into four or six burgers.
• Dust the burgers lightly with flour. Fry them in the pan in which you fried the onions, adding a little more oil, if necessary, for 3–4 minutes on each side.
• The burgers are delicious hot or cold. Serve them on their own with a salad, or in a traditional bun with raw onion, crunchy iceberg lettuce, and ketchup.

★ **vegetable oil, for frying**
★ **1 large onion, finely chopped**
★ **12oz/375g chuck steak or shin of beef, all fat removed, minced**
★ **8oz/250g carrot, finely grated**
1 tbsp whole wheat breadcrumbs
★ **1 tbsp chopped fresh mint**
★ **1 tbsp chopped fresh parsley**
flour, for dusting

indian kidney beans

Serves 2

This delicious dish is fabulous served with basmati rice. It can, of course, be made with dried beans, but they must be soaked overnight and boiled hard for 10 minutes then cooked more gently for another 20 before you can use them – too much fuss, perhaps, for most working parents!

• Melt the butter in a heavy-bottomed frying pan. Add the onions and fry gently until golden. Add the garlic and pepper and fry over a medium heat until the pepper is cooked. Make sure the garlic does not become too dark. Add the beans with half their liquid, the cilantro, garam masala, and salt. Cover the pan and cook for about five minutes.

★ 3 tbsp butter
★ 1 onion, chopped
★ 1 clove garlic, chopped
★ 1 green bell pepper, seeded and chopped
★ 13oz/400g canned red kidney beans
★ 1–2 tbsp chopped cilantro
1 tsp garam masala
salt

oliver's pizza

Makes 2

These pizzas can be frozen before wrapping to be stored in the freezer. If they are to be cooked directly from the freezer, allow about 7 minutes' extra cooking time.

• To make the crusts, put the flours, salt, and yeast in a warm, dry bowl and mix well. Make a well in the center, add the water and olive oil, and mix to a dough. On a lightly floured surface knead the dough for 3 minutes, or until it feels firm and springy. Put the dough in a clean, warm bowl, cover with plastic wrap or a clean dish towel, and let it rise in a warm place for up to 2 hours.

• Meanwhile, make a tomato sauce for the topping. Heat the oil in a saucepan, add the onion and garlic, and fry over a gentle heat till soft and translucent. Add the tomatoes and the marjoram or oregano, crushing the tomatoes roughly with the back of a wooden spoon. Cook until the sauce has thickened and reduced a little.

• Preheat the oven to 375°F/190°C. Take the dough from the bowl and divide it in two. Roll out each piece of dough to a 12in/30cm circle. Put in two oiled pizza pans and brush the surfaces with oil. Cover with slices of mozzarella, then some tomato sauce. Sprinkle grated cheese over the tops. Bake the pizzas in the oven for about 20 minutes.

For the pizza bases:
2 cups/250g bread flour
★ 2 cups/250g whole wheat flour
2 tsp salt
2 x ¼oz (6g) packages dried yeast
1¼ cups/300ml tepid water
(1 part boiling to 2 parts cold)
4 tbsp olive oil

For the topping:
★ 2 tbsp olive oil
★ 1 onion, finely chopped
★ 1 clove garlic, crushed
★ 8oz/250g canned tomatoes
★ fresh marjoram or good pinch of dried oregano
★ 3½oz/100g mozzarella or other firm soft cheese, sliced
★ 2 tbsp grated cheddar or other hard cheese

desserts

Children need no persuading to eat sweet things. Choose any of the tempting desserts here and you will be giving your youngsters nutritious food that they will eat with pleasure.

fruit dipped in chocolate sauce

★ = superfood

Serves 4

Choose your children's favorite fruit for this fondue – apples, pears, grapes, strawberries, peaches, tangerine segments, chunks of pineapple, bananas, melon – and use organic chocolate, if possible. Have plenty of wooden skewers handy for dipping the fruit into the chocolate.

• Cut large fruits into chunks, if appropriate, and put all the fruit in a bowl or on a large platter.

• Break the chocolate into pieces and put it in a bowl set over a pan of hot, but not boiling water. Let it melt. Keep hot in a fondue pot or over a tea light while the children are dipping fruit into it.

★ **fresh fruit, washed and chilled for 2–3 hours**

8–10oz/250–300g bittersweet chocolate

Illustrated right

creamy fruit tart

Serves 6

• Heat the oven to 425°F/220°C. Lightly grease a 12 in/30cm springform pan. Wash, dry, halve, and stone the fruit.

• Roll out the pastry on a lightly floured surface and use to line the pan. Lay the prepared fruit lightly on the pastry, cut sides down.

• Beat the eggs in a bowl, add the crème fraîche and sugar, and beat together until smooth. Pour the mixture over the fruit. Sprinkle extra sugar on top.

• Bake in the oven for about 30 minutes, or until the top is lightly golden.

★ **8 large ripe plums, apricots, or small peaches**

8oz/250g puff pastry, thawed if frozen

★ **2 eggs**

★ **1 cup/200ml crème fraîche**

2 tbsp superfine sugar, plus extra for sprinkling

½ tsp vanilla extract

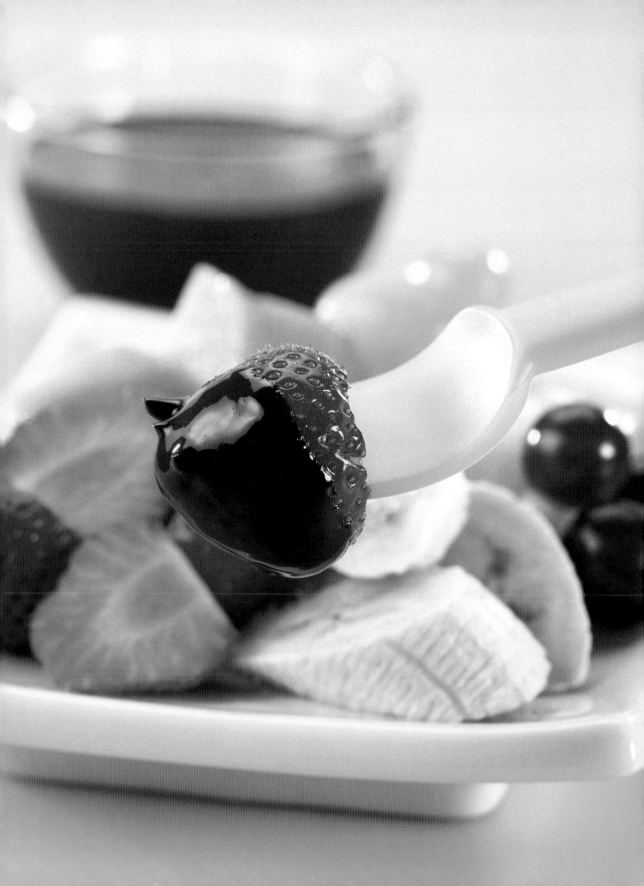

summer pudding

★ = superfood

Serves 4

Classic Summer Pudding is made with white bread and much more white sugar than this version calls for. But the pudding works just as well with whole wheat bread, and the delicious fruity taste comes through much more sharply when it is not overwhelmed by sugar. You may find you like even less. Make the pudding at least six hours before it is going to be served.

• Wash the fruit and put it all into a large saucepan along with the sugar. Set the pan over a very low heat for 2–3 minutes until the sugar melts and the juices begin to run. Set aside.

• Use five slices of the bread to line a 2lb/1kg serving dish, making sure there are no gaps which could spoil the dessert's appearance. Add the fruit, reserving a half of a cup of the juice. Place the remaining slice of bread over the pudding, then put a plate on top with a weight on it to press it down into the dish. Chill the dessert for at least 6 hours.

• To serve, invert the dish over a serving plate so that the pudding slides onto the middle of it. Pour the reserved juice and serve, on its own or with Greek yogurt or a little crème fraîche.

- ★ 12oz/375g raspberries
- ★ 6oz/180g red currants
- ★ 2oz/60g blackberries or blueberries
- ⅓ cup/60g soft brown sugar
- ★ 6 thin slices whole wheat bread, crusts removed
- ★ crème fraîche or Greek yogurt, for serving

upside-down pudding

Serves 4

• Heat the oven to 350°F/180°C. Lightly grease a 9in/23cm cake pan.

• Cream together 8 tbsp/125g softened butter and the superfine sugar. Beat in the eggs, one at a time, until the mixture is light and fluffy. Fold in the flour.

• Melt the remaining butter and pour it all over the bottom of the prepared pan. Sprinkle on the brown sugar evenly. Arrange the fruits neatly in an attractive flower-like pattern in the pan, decorating the pattern with the cherries. Try not to leave gaps.

• Spread the batter over the top of the fruit. Bake on the middle shelf of the oven for 45 minutes, or until a skewer inserted into the center of the cake comes out clean. Turn the pudding out onto a plate. Serve it while warm with whipped cream, fromage frais, or vanilla ice cream.

- ★ 10 tbsp/150g butter, softened, plus extra for greasing
- ½ cup/125g superfine sugar
- ★ 2 eggs
- 1 cup/125g self-rising flour, sifted
- ⅓ cup/60g soft brown sugar
- ★ 13oz/400g fresh fruit, such as pineapple, apricots, pears, weighed after peeling and cutting into chunks
- ★ a few cherries
- ★ whipped cream, fromage frais or vanilla ice cream, for serving

ginger fruit pudding

Serves 4

• Heat the oven to 350°F/180°C. Lightly butter a 5 cups/1.2 liter capacity deep ovenproof dish.

• Sift the flour, cinnamon, nutmeg, ginger, baking soda, and sugar into a bowl, tipping the bran left in the sifter into the dry ingredients. Mix in the egg.

• Melt the butter in a small saucepan and add the molasses to warm through. Add this to the flour-and-egg mixture, then pour in the milk. Using a balloon whisk, mix thoroughly so there are no lumps. Stir in the raisins and preserved ginger.

• Pour the mixture into the prepared dish. Bake in the oven for 30–35 minutes. Do not overcook and don't worry if it subsides a bit in the middle; this gives a nice sticky center to the pudding.

• Serve hot with chilled whipped cream. You can add some of the syrup from the preserved ginger to the whipped cream, if you wish.

★ 1 cup/125g whole wheat self-rising flour
★ 1 pinch salt
★ 2 tsp cinnamon
★ ½ tsp grated nutmeg
★ 1 tsp ground ginger
1 tsp baking soda
½ cup/125g soft dark brown sugar
★ 1 egg
★ 4 tbsp/60g butter
⅓ cup/90g molasses
★ 1¼ cups/300ml milk
★ 2oz/60g golden raisins
★ 4 pieces (more if you like) preserved ginger), chopped
★ whipped cream, to serve

blackberry & apple crumble

Serves 4

• Heat the oven to 350°F/180°C. Butter a baking dish well.

• Peel, core, and slice the apples, wash the blackberries and put both kinds of fruit into the baking dish. Add the sugar and sprinkle with the lemon juice.

• To make the topping, put the flour and brown sugar in a bowl and rub in the butter until the mixture resembles coarse breadcrumbs. Mix in the nuts. Sprinkle the topping over the fruit.

• Put the dish on a baking sheet and bake in the oven for 45 minutes to 1 hour, or until the topping becomes crisp.

★ 1lb/500g apples
★ 1lb/500g blackberries
1 tbsp brown sugar
★ 1 tsp lemon juice

For the topping:
★ 1½ cups/180g whole wheat flour
½ cup/90g brown sugar
★ 6 tbsp/90g butter, diced
★ ¾ cup/90g chopped mixed nuts

pancakes

★ = superfood

Makes about 8

★ **3 eggs**
★ **1¼ cup/150g whole wheat flour**
★ **1 cup/250ml milk**
1 tsp brown sugar
★ **butter, for cooking**

Pancakes are fun for everyone in the family to join in making – men tend to take over tossing them. Even young children can mix and make pancakes successfully – though perhaps without the tossing!

• Beat the eggs lightly and whisk in the flour, milk, and sugar. Leave the batter in the refrigerator for at least 30 minutes (or up to 24 hours, if necessary).

• When you're ready to make the pancakes, melt a little butter in a small omelette pan. When it is frothing, add about 4 tablespoons of the batter and cook for about 1 minute on each side – it is time to turn the pancake when little bubbles have appeared all over the surface. Keep the pancakes warm in the oven until everybody is ready – or serve them as soon as they're cooked. This should be a noisy, messy meal!

• Serve with a selection of accompaniments: lemon juice, sugar, apple purée, strawberries, or raspberries stewed for just a couple of minutes to get their juices running, sugar-free fruit purée, or ice cream.

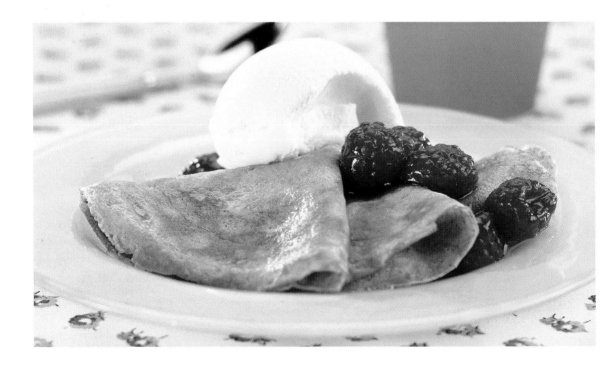

real rice pudding

Serves 4

This has been a kids' treat forever and totally unlike anything you can buy ready-made in the supermarket. A delicious source of worthwhile calories and calcium, rice pudding can be served with any cooked fruit, apple purée or fruit preserves.

• Heat the oven to 300°F/150°C. Use a little of the butter to grease a shallow ovenproof dish.
• Put the rice, milk, and sugar in the dish and stir well. Dot with tiny bits of the remaining butter and add freshly grated nutmeg.
• Transfer the dish to the oven. Bake for 15 minutes, then stir the pudding gently. Bake for another 15 minutes and stir again. Cook for another $1^1/_2$ hours until there is a crisp brown skin on top of the pudding.

★ 3 tbsp/45g butter
★ 3 tbsp rice
★ 2½ cups/600ml whole milk
2 tbsp brown sugar
★ pinch of nutmeg

stewed apple with mascarpone

Serves 4

This wonderful variation on traditional stewed apples has the added benefit of protein and calcium from mascarpone cheese. Depending on your children's taste, you can add a sprig of mint, a few cloves, or both, while the apples are stewing.

• Put the water into a saucepan. Add the sugar and heat gently until the sugar has dissolved.
• Add the apple slices to the sugar mixture, cooking very gently. When the apples have cooked to a smooth purée, fold in the mascarpone.
• Put in individual dishes and chill in the refrigerator.

¼ cup/60ml water
2 tbsp/30g superfine sugar
★ 1lb/500g cooking apples, such as Granny Smiths, peeled, cored and sliced
★ 8oz/250g mascarpone cheese

prune purée

Serves 4

This simple dessert is super-rich in antioxidants and also has a little iron and lots of fiber.

• Put the prunes in a bowl, cover with boiling water, and let them soak overnight. Next day, remove the pits from the prunes and chop the prunes coarsely.
• Put the remaining ingredients in a bowl and whisk until the egg whites stiffens. Fold in the prunes and refrigerate for 2 hours. Serve with natural yogurt mixed with peel from the second lemon, if desired, and a pinch of allspice.

★ 1lb/500g prunes
★ juice of 2 unwaxed lemons
★ peel of one of the lemons
3 tbsp/45g light brown granulated sugar
★ 3 egg whites from guaranteed salmonella-free, free-range eggs (because the eggs are ucooked)
★ yogurt and allspice, to serve

delicious drinks

Children need to **drink a lot of liquids**. Fluids help avoid common problems like constipation. Avoid high-sugar, high-caffeine soft drinks, and use a juicer or blender to make the **great beverages** here

kiwi surprise

Serves 1–2

Illustrated top

This is an immunity-boosting glass of brain power which children love.
• Juice all the ingredients in a juicer.

★ **4 carrots**
★ **1 apple, quartered**
★ **1 kiwi fruit**

berry delight

Serves 1–2

Illustrated middle

Here is a drink that is high in energy, bursting with vitamin C, and full of the most powerful immunity-boosting and cancer-protective plant chemicals.
• Put all the ingredients in a blender and process until smooth.

★ **2/3 cup/150g natural yogurt**
★ **1¼ cups/300ml milk (full-fat for the under 5s)**
★ **fresh or frozen berries – a mixture or all one variety, such as strawberries, blueberries, and raspberries**
a handful of ice cubes

coconut crush

Serves 2

Illustrated bottom

Older children will love the tropical smell and taste of this highly nutritious drink. It is especially good for girls because of its high calcium content and the phytoestrogens in the soy milk.
• Put all the ingredients in a blender and process until smooth.

★ **1¼ cups/300ml soy milk**
2/3 cup/150g coconut milk
★ **2/3 cup/150g frozen natural yogurt**
½ tsp ground cinnamon
¼ tsp ground cloves
a handful of ice cubes

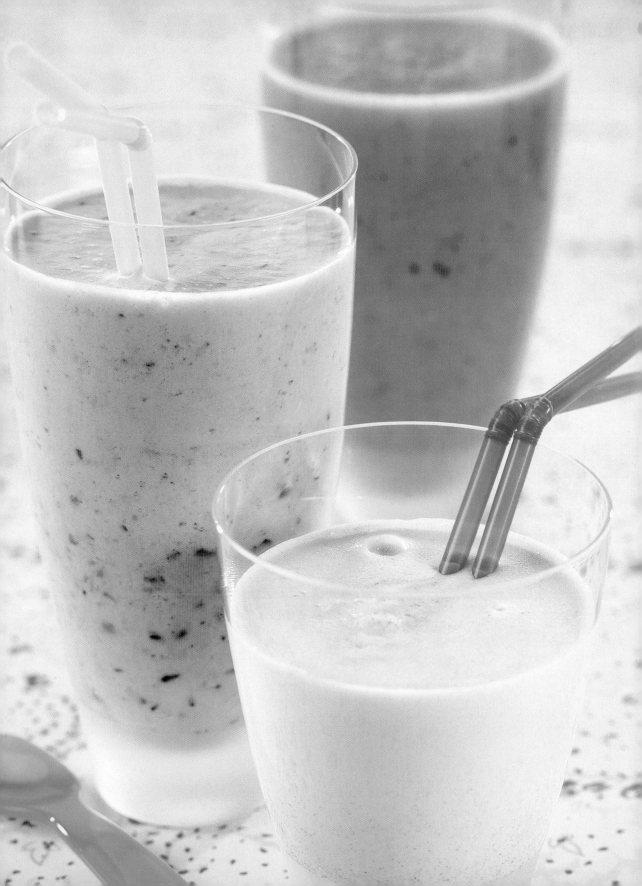

pear power

Serves 1–2

Few people realize the nutritional value of a ripe pear. This drink provides a rich supply of natural sugars – just the thing for instant energy.
• Juice all the ingredients in a juicer.

★ 4 pears, quartered
★ 2 slices fresh pineapple
★ 2 apples, quartered
★ 12 grapes, red or green

tomatoes plus

Serves 1–2

This mind-and-body juice is super-rich in minerals to invigorate tired young muscles, and full of calming essential oils from the basil to revive the flagging mind and spirit.
• Juice the tomatoes, carrot, celery, and basil in a juicer. Stir in the lemon juice, Worcestershire sauce, and freshly ground black pepper.

★ 4 large ripe plum tomatoes
★ 1 carrot, roughly chopped
★ 1 stick celery
★ handful of basil leaves
★ juice of 1/2 lemon
dash of Worcestershire sauce
black pepper

nutty apple juice

Serves 1–2

This may sound like a kids' party treat, but it's also a real energy-boosting, nutritious smoothie. Instantly available calories from the fruit sugar in the apples mixed with the slower release calories in bananas make this suitable before sustained physical activity. Make sure you select one of the "healthy" peanut butters - without added salt.
• Juice the apples in a juicer, add the bananas and peanut butter and blend together.

★ 6 apples, quartered
★ 2 bananas
★ 1 tbsp smooth unsalted peanut butter

jungle juice

Serves 1–2

Juice the mango and passionfruit in a juicer and blend with the yogurt and milk.

1 mango, peeled and stoned
2 passionfruit, flesh and seeds scooped from skins
★ 2/3 cup/150g frozen natural yogurt
★ 11/4 cups/300ml whole milk

dark fruit drink

Serves 1–2

Prunes are famed for their gentle laxative action, but because of their high potassium content they're good for maintaining normal blood pressure, too.
• Juice the apples and pears in a juicer. Purée the prunes in a blender, then add the juice, lecithin, and molasses and purée everything together.

★ 4 apples, quartered
★ 4 ripe pears, quartered
★ 6 prunes, soaked and pitted
2 tsp lecithin granules
2 tsp molasses

lemonade mix

Serves 4–6

Make your own lemonade and avoid all the chemical additives, flavorings, and colorings in the commercial drinks. The small amount of effort will be hugely repaid in taste and health benefits.

• Peel the lemons, leaving as much pith as possible on the fruit. Squeeze the juice from the peeled lemons into a large bowl and add the sugar.

• Put the peel and water into a saucepan, bring to a boil, and simmer for 3 minutes. Strain the liquid into the juice, stirring until all the sugar has dissolved.

• Pour into a jar with a tightly fitting lid and keep in the refrigerator. To drink the lemonade, dilute it to taste with ice-cold water.

★ 6 unwaxed lemons
2 1/4 cups/500g granulated sugar
2 1/2 cups/1.2 liters water

sesame smoothie

Serves 1–2

This calcium- and energy-rich smoothie makes a great after-school reviver.

• Put the yogurt, tahini and ice cubes in a blender and process until smooth. Pour into glasses and sprinkle the sesame seeds on top.

★ 1 1/4 cups/300ml natural yogurt
★ 1 tbsp tahini
a handful of ice cubes
★ 1 tsp sesame seeds

tropical delight

Serves 1–2

Put the mango, pineapple, ginger and lime in a juicer and juice well together. Blend the juice with the yogurt and the ice cubes for a delicious fruit tea.

1 mango, peeled and pitted
★ 1 pineapple, top removed, cut into chunks
★ 1in/2.5cm piece fresh ginger
★ 1 lime, peeled and sliced
★ 2/3 cup/150g natural yogurt
a handful of ice cubes

b plus

Serves 1-2

This delicious drink is wonderfully high in B vitamins.

• Juice the tomatoes, celery, and parsley in a juicer, then blend with the remaining ingredients.

★ 6 tomatoes, quartered
★ 2 sticks celery, chopped
★ handful of parsley, with stalks
★ 2/3 cup/150g natural yogurt
★ 1/2 cup/125g cottage cheese
2 tsp brewer's yeast
Worcestershire sauce, to taste

instant good food

You're **home late** and there isn't time to make the meal you planned. Or your children have just come home bringing some **hungry friends**. Or the pizza place was **overcrowded** so you decided to eat at home instead. Or you all got home **ravenous** from a day's outing and your mind is a complete blank, even with a well-filled refrigerator, pantry, and freezer.

Here are suggestions for moments like this. They range from quick snacks to full-blown meals, with some ideas for quick healthy desserts, too. None of them is complicated: some don't even need a recipe. And some are from the Recipes section, with page references to help you find them quickly. Frozen herbs come into their own here: a teaspoon of chopped chives or parsley scooped out of a freezer container can make a huge difference to the appeal of these meals. And if you also have frozen beans, green peas, broccoli, or spinach, you can turn a snack into a healthy meal.

Baked beans on toast with sliced tomatoes on top.

Oven-baked beans Heat the oven to moderately hot. Drain and thoroughly rinse a can of red kidney or cannellini beans. Heat a little oil in a saucepan, add the beans, and toss. Turn the heat down very low, cover and gently heat the beans through for 5 minutes. Drizzle a little extra-virgin olive oil over thick slices of whole wheat bread or halved rolls, spread a little mustard on them, put on a baking sheet, and top with the heated beans. Cover the beans with slices of tomato, top with grated cheddar cheese, and put in the oven for 10 minutes or until the cheese is melting and bubbly.

Onions and beans Melt a teaspoon of butter in a pan and gently fry a sliced onion in it until soft; add a dash of lemon juice. Add baked beans, toss, lower the heat, cover, and let the beans heat through. Add black pepper and parsley and serve on buttered whole wheat toast.

Canned tuna can be turned into many quick, delicious, easy meals.

Tuna and beans Flake canned tuna into rinsed and drained canned white beans (or borlotti or red kidney beans) and dress with plenty of olive oil, lemon juice, and seasoning. Garnish with onion rings, tomato slices, and parsley or chives.

Tuna and potato salad Boil and peel small new potatoes; put them into a salad bowl with flaked tuna, sliced onion rings, and a few black olives. Make a dressing with olive oil, lemon juice, black pepper, chopped garlic, mayonnaise, and a touch of anchovy paste. Mix well and pour over the potatoes while still hot. Toss gently.

Tuna-egg salad Hard-boil one egg per person. Arrange the shelled and halved eggs on a dish; mix a well-drained can of tuna with mayonnaise and cover the eggs with it. Serve with plenty of crusty bread.

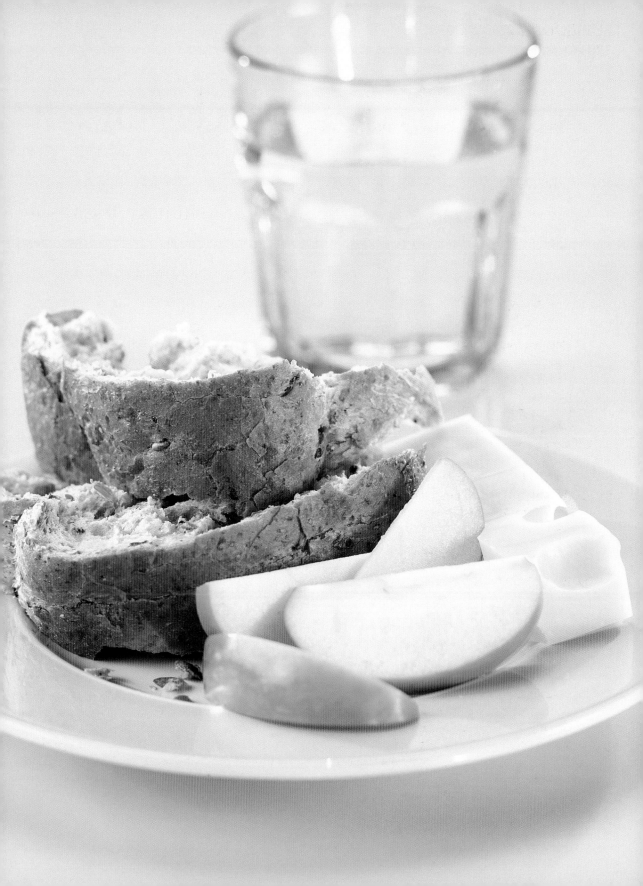

Tuna and corn salad

Put some frozen corn in a pan with enough water to cover, bring to a boil, simmer for 2–3 minutes, then drain. Add chunks of tomato and beets, chopped scallions, and a can of drained, flaked tuna. Make a creamy dressing with olive oil, lemon juice, seasoning, a teaspoonful of mustard, and a dollop of mayonnaise. Pour over the salad and toss gently.

Whole wheat bread

can be used in many ways. Cut whole wheat rolls in half, toast them, then drizzle the cut halves with a little olive oil. Top with lightly seasoned, large slices of tomatoes and slices of mozzarella, and drizzle pesto sauce over all.

Pizza-style bread

Toast one side of halved whole wheat rolls, thick slices of whole wheat bread, whole wheat pitas, or lengths of baguette. Drizzle olive oil over the untoasted sides, top with slices of tomato and season with dried oregano and a little freshly ground pepper. Grate cheddar cheese on top and put under a hot broiler until the cheese bubbles.

Mushrooms on toast with crumbly cheese

uses mushrooms, any hard cheese, and bacon (see page 153).

Granny Smith's Welsh rarebit

uses Cheddar cheese, cream, and apples (see page 155).

Bread and cheese bake

Preheat the oven to hot. For four people, butter four slices of whole wheat bread and cut into squares. Finely chop an onion. Grate a 6oz/180g piece of hard cheese. Lightly butter a pie dish, and put a layer of bread squares on the bottom. Add half the onion, and top with half the cheese. Repeat the bread, onion and cheese layers. Then beat 4 eggs in 2½ cups/ 600ml milk, season them with salt and pepper, and pour the eggs over the layered bread and cheese. Bake in the preheated oven for about 30 minutes until golden brown.

Plowman's lunch or supper

needs a decent cheese, and a few scallions. Serve the cheese with some interesting bread, defrosted if frozen and then warmed in the oven.

Coleslaw

can be prepared quickly. Shred a chunk of white cabbage, a couple of carrots, and a crisp apple; add a dressing made with mayonnaise thinned down slightly with a little olive oil and lemon juice. Garnish with parsley or chives.

Chunks of mild cheese

– Gouda, Jarlsberg, Emmenthal, or a mild Cheddar – served with oatcakes, a glass of milk, and an apple adds up to a quick and nutritious bedtime snack for small children.

Eggs

are a good start for many a sustaining snack. You can poach them, scramble them, make them into an omelette, or just boil them, and serve with toast. Some variations on the eggs theme:

Spanish omelette

is an excellent and quick dish, needing only a salad to make it a satisfying meal (see page 145 for recipe).

Eggs and spinach mornay

Preheat the oven to moderately hot. Hard-boil an egg for each person. Defrost a package of spinach; mix in a teaspoon of butter and freshly grated nutmeg; put the mixture into a baking dish, top with the hard-boiled eggs sliced in two lengthwise, cover with Sauce Mornay (see below), top with grated cheese, and bake in the oven for 10–15 minute.

To make enough Sauce Mornay for four, heat 1¼ cups/300ml milk. In a nonstick pan melt 2 tablespoons butter and add 2 tablespoons whole wheat flour (or half white and half whole wheat), and stir until the mixture is smooth. Add the milk, a little at a time, stirring to keep the sauce smooth. Add 2 tablespoons grated hard cheese, a heaping teaspoon French mustard, a little pepper, and stir again. Reduce the heat and cook for 5–10 minutes, stirring occasionally.

Potato omelette is a simpler version of the classic Spanish tortilla. Peel 2–3 potatoes, grate, rinse, and dry in a dish towel. Beat together 3 or 4 eggs, add a tablespoon of milk, the grated potatoes, chopped parsley or chives, and seasoning. Melt a little butter in a non-stick frying pan, add the mixture, lower the heat, cover, and cook for 10 minutes. Flip the omelette over, cook for a little longer, and serve with a salad or green vegetable.

Baked potatoes For every two people, bake one big potato well pierced with a fork in a very hot oven for up to an hour: the potatoes are cooked when they give and feel slightly soft. When they're done, halve them, scoop out most of the flesh into a bowl, mash it with a little butter, milk, or cream cheese, and refill the potato skins. Make a hollow in the middle of each filling, break an egg into it, cover with grated cheese, and return to the oven until the cheese is golden and bubbly and the egg has set.

Cooked rice is a good stir-fry basic. Stir-fry sliced and diced vegetables, such as carrots, onions, leeks, cabbage, zucchini, and tomatoes, in a wok. Add the cold cooked rice, a cupful of hot vegetable stock and simmer, covered, for 20 minutes.

Rice croquettes also use cooked rice. Add grated cheese, chopped parsley, and a beaten egg to the rice and form it into croquettes. Dust with seasoned flour and fry.

A sausage dinner Cook some peeled potatoes in boiling salted water. Broil some link sausages. Heat some olive oil in a frying pan and fry a couple of onions cut into thick slices. When the potatoes and sausages are done, cut them into chunks and put them in a serving bowl with the drained fried onion. Add a little more oil to the pan in which the onions were fried plus a teaspoon of mustard and a dash of vinegar, swirl around to mix, and pour over the sausages and potatoes. Chopped celery would be a good, crunchy addition.

Cottage cheese makes a good foundation for a warm summer supper. Add to it chunks of cucumber, tomato, green pepper, some onion rings, and black olives. Dress with plenty of olive oil, lemon juice, fresh herbs, and seasonings for a variation on Greek salad. Add feta cheese to make it authentic.

Pasta, the original fast food, is ever-popular. Turn to pages 176-177 for some excellent sauces, including a quick tomato sauce, which can be prepared as you need them, or made in advance and kept in the refrigerator for several days.

Greek yogurt is a great standby for quick and healthy desserts. Start with some creamy thick Greek yogurt and stir flaked almonds or chopped nuts into it with a drizzle of honey. Or stir in some puréed fruit, crushed strawberries, and raspberries, or a spoonful of a no added sugar fruit spread. Or defrost a package of frozen forest fruits, heat through, adding slices of peach or nectarine or any other fresh fruit available, and serve with dollops of yogurt.

In summertime, cottage cheese makes a lovely dessert: serve it with fresh fruit, such as chunks of peach or nectarine, a few strawberries, or a handful of grapes, and a little orange juice and finely grated orange zest.

Pancakes can be a fun family occasion as well as a memorable dessert: see page 190 for a good basic recipe along with plenty of ideas for serving them.

And everyone loves baked apples. Core and slice them and place in a thick layer on a buttered shallow baking pan. Pour the juice of a couple of lemons over them, a sprinkling of brown sugar, and some small pieces of butter. Add a spoonful of apple juice, white wine, or water and put in a very hot oven until the apple slices are soft and gilded. Serve with thick yogurt or fresh cream.

special problems

Foods children eat contribute not only to the quality of their general health but also to their susceptibility to numerous food-related disorders. While the wrong foods can be a cause of eating disorders and other problems, switching to healthier foods can alleviate many of them.

food & disorders

Never before have the ingredients for a **healthy** and **delicious** diet been so **widely available** as they are to families today. Walk into any supermarket and you will see a cornucopia of **wonderful foods** from the world over. Despite this, diet-connected problems are increasing among children.

One of the reasons for this is that millions of children in the Western world live on poor and extremely limited diets featuring chiefly high-fat, high-sugar convenience foods that supply abundant calories but disastrously few of the nutrients required for growing children. Deficiencies in the B vitamins and in minerals, such as zinc, magnesium, and iron, can not only affect normal growth and development but also adversely affect the nervous system and crucial areas of brain function.

These deficiencies are increasingly common in today's children, with anemia (caused by iron deficiency), scurvy (caused by a lack of vitamin C), and rickets (caused by a lack of vitamin D) all showing significant rises, especially among children living in inner cities.

children and food-related disorders

Parents today are encountering a whole new range of childhood food-related disorders for which there is no swift medical fix, and, often, no real medical understanding either.

Allergic problems have become much more common, with the incidence of conditions such as asthma and eczema increasing inexorably. More and more children, boys as well as girls, are developing eating disorders such as anorexia. And attention deficit hyperactivity disorder (ADHD) affects all too many children in the West.

Many factors are known to contribute to the increase in these and other problems, stress and environmental pollution among them. But many careful studies suggest that what children eat, as well as what is missing from their diets, can be vital contributory causes.

the benefits of eating organic foods

A major problem is the numerous pesticides used in food production, traces of which turn up in many foods, with unknown consequences for children's health and development. Dr. Vyvyan Howard, a leading fetal and infant toxicology expert at the University of Liverpool in the UK, is emphatic in his advice: "One of the most positive things we can do is eat organic food. This considerably reduces the 'body burden' of toxic chemicals in both parent and child."

The right diet, rich in natural, organic foods, certainly will not solve all these problems. But by feeding your children good, simple, healthy food from day one, and by teaching them the basic principles of good nutrition, you will certainly avoid the worst of them.

If, despite all your efforts, problems do arise and a doctor is unable to help, consider seeking the advice of a trained, qualified, and registered complementary therapist, such as a homeopath, naturopath, or herbalist (see Resources, page 214).

allergies

An allergy is an inappropriate response from the body's immune system to a substance that is not normally harmful. The immune system is a complex mechanism which helps the body combat infections. It does this by identifying "foreign bodies" and then mobilizing the white cells to destroy them.

Sometimes, the immune system mistakes an innocent substance for an invader. The white cells over-react, producing large quantities of the chemical histamine and the symptoms of asthma, hay fever, eczema, and all the other allergic symptoms that plague so many people.

As our society has become more affluent, so the number of people suffering from allergies has risen. Our fresh air is polluted by traffic fumes; our homes are centrally heated, with double-paned windows and wall-to-wall carpeting, to the delight of the house-dust mite; our work places are often sealed boxes without a single opening window so they are too hot in the winter and overly air-conditioned in the summer.

identifying signs of allergic reaction

The other effect of affluence is the world-wide food production network, making it possible for children to eat favorite foods through the whole twelve months of the year, and in ever increasing quantities. The more they eat the same foods, the more likely it is that allergies will develop. In fish-eating countries, fish allergies are more common; in countries where dairy products are a substantial part of the diet, allergy to these is more common.

The instant reactions which produce large quantities of histamine also produce instant symptoms. Blotchy skin, hives, swollen mouth, and throat, streaming eyes, paroxysms of sneezing, are all immediately obvious. But it's also possible for food allergies to be delayed because killer T-cells, part of the body's immune-system defense mechanism, react to non-protein substances like nickel and other heavy metals, cosmetics, perfumes, and even food additives, setting off an allergic response up to 48 hours later. This makes the offenders difficult to identify. Common culprits are citrus fruits, garlic, mangoes, celery, and even carrots. Chemicals added to food for coloring, flavoring, or preserving can work in the same way.

Another example of non-acute food allergy is coeliac disease where sufferers are allergic to the gluten in wheat and other grains. Impaired nutrient absorption, weight loss, and general malaise result.

allergy or intolerance?

There is a problem about deciding whether a child is suffering from food allergy (a reaction to allergens) or food intolerance (a condition for which allergic antibodies are not responsible). In the past decade there has been enormous media coverage of food allergies and a mushrooming boom in dubious allergy clinics and allergy-testing methods. There is also a plethora of pseudo-scientific mumbo jumbo which has made huge numbers of people obsessed with what they eat, drink, breathe, wear, and even where they live.

About half the world's population does not produce the enzyme needed to digest milk (see page 204), so milk intolerance is widespread, and common in children. Coffee, tea, cocoa, chocolate, cheese, beer, sausages, canned foods, red wine, wheat, and tomatoes are all foods that the body may not tolerate.

Migraine, asthma, eczema, urticaria (hives), irritable bowel syndrome, colitis, Crohn's disease, hay fever, and rheumatoid arthritis are just some of the illnesses which can involve food allergy or intolerance. They may all respond to the right dietary changes. Unfortunately, the only way to be certain that you are making appropriate dietary modifications to relieve the problem is to follow a lengthy and quite laborious exclusion diet.

It is essential, particularly when dealing with children, that any major change in eating habits is monitored by a doctor or an expert nutritionist. It is not uncommon for allergy enthusiasts to recommend diets that are so restricted that their patients become severely malnourished, weak, and very ill. If a child has a severe "anaphylactic" allergy, which could be very serious, your physician will provide you with an emergency injection kit should the worst happen and the child unwittingly eats a peanut or a few sesame seeds, or gets stung by a bee or a wasp.

nutrition and allergies

While there has been little scientific research to confirm the theory, there is evidence that increasing consumption of some nutrients, either from foods or supplements, can lessen allergic reactions. B vitamins, particularly niacin and pantothenic acid, are thought to help with respiratory infections, nasal congestion, and hay fever. Vitamin B_6 may reduce sensitivity to monosodium glutamate. Vitamin B_{12} is believed to reduce post-nasal drip and sensitivity to the sulfite preservatives. The essential fatty acids and omega-3 fatty acids in evening primrose oil and fish oils, along with magnesium, have been shown to help reduce the allergic reaction in atopic (childhood) eczema.

foods that cause allergies

Several foods are recognized as being common causes of allergic reactions among children. Some of these, such as berries, are seasonal and eaten less frequently; others are year-round basic superfoods.

If a child gets the occasional bout of something that looks like a rash for no obvious reason, or even red itchy patches that fade within a few hours, it is sensible to suspect a food allergy and to think back to what he or she has eaten in the past day. A common cause of such reactions among children, especially in the summer months, is berries, with strawberries near the top of the list.

Severe reactions are most likely from nuts, seeds, fish, shellfish, and eggs. Less severe chronic symptoms are normally caused by milk and milk products, soy-based products, food additives (except for asthmatics who may react severely to some of these), and gluten-containing cereals, which include wheat, oats, and barley. Other things that children may consume frequently when the summer comes, and which are common allergens, are carbonated drinks, pineapple, cherries, and plums.

If your child is strongly allergic to any foods, you will soon know what they are, but slight reactions can sometimes go unrecognized.

References to the most common allergy-causing foods occur throughout this book. Here, their causes and symptoms are summarized.

Cow's milk and its dairy products head the list of foods that may cause allergic reactions among children. The reaction is to a protein in the milk. Symptoms include diarrhea, vomiting, colic in babies, and abdominal pain in older children, eczema, sinus, and respiratory problems.

Babies and children allergic to cow's milk should be treated under the supervision of a doctor or nutritionist. If breast-feeding is not an option, babies may be given a hypoallergenic or soy-based formula milk. Older children may need to be fed a dairy-free diet.

Lactose intolerance is caused by a lack in the system of a digestive enzyme, lactase, which normally digests lactose, the sugar in cow's milk. In Western countries, where most people retain lactase in the intestine throughout life, lactose intolerance is usually caused by gastrointestinal bacteria or a virus damaging the gut and is a temporary problem.

Wheat is a fairly common cause of problems in young children, probably because of the great amount of wheat-based foods eaten today. If your child has vague symptoms of digestive discomfort, lethargy, irregular bowel function, and general malaise, for which no other specific cause can be found, it is worth trying a week or two without any wheat whatsover. Substitute rice cakes, rye crispbread, pumpernickel, products made with buckwheat, chickpea, rice, or potato flour, or any other non-wheat product.

If there is a problem with gluten allergy, as in celiac disease, all gluten-containing cereals, including wheat, oats, barley, rye, must be avoided. No babies should have gluten foods until six months, or up to a year if there is a history of wheat or gluten intolerance in the family.

Nuts and seeds, particularly peanuts, but also walnuts, pecans, and cashews, can cause rashes, asthma, and eczema.

In severe cases – fortunately very rare – nuts can cause potentially fatal anaphylactic shock. If there is any history of food allergy in a child's family, nutritionists recommend that the child should not be given nuts in any form until he is at least five years old. If there is no history of allergy, children may be given an easily eaten form of peanuts, such as smooth peanut butter, from the age of 18 months. Whole nuts should never be given to children under three years old because they could choke on them.

Eggs may cause rashes, swelling, and stomach upsets, asthma, and childhood eczema (atopic eczema). Since the reaction is often to the egg white rather than the whole egg, foods that should be avoided include desserts such as mousses and meringues, as well as cakes, mayonnaise, and ice cream.

Fish, both fresh (such as cod and sole) and smoked (smoked salmon, haddock, and trout) can cause skin rashes, stomach upsets, nausea, and migraine. Shellfish, both crustaceans and mollusks, can cause severe and prolonged stomach upsets as well as the migraine and nausea associated with fish allergies.

dealing with allergy foods

The only treatment for food allergy in children is abstinence, and the way to find out what you should avoid giving your child is to follow an exclusion diet, such as the one set out on the opposite page.

This exclusion diet may look difficult, but it only needs to be followed rigorously for about two weeks, after which foods may be added back, provided you keep a record. You will soon be able to build a list of foods which your child can tolerate and eliminate the others.

Stick rigidly to the diet for at least two weeks and keep a diary to pinpoint bad reactions. After two weeks things should improve. If they do not, food allergy or intolerance is probably not the problem and you should get further medical help.

exclusion diet for allergies

The diet is set out in two columns. In the "not allowed" column are all those foods that a child should not eat in any form for the first two weeks of the diet. The list may seem rather long, but a glance at the "allowed" column will show you such a good range of foods that, with a bit of careful planning, a child need never notice that he is being deprived of any favorite foods.

Foods for the first two weeks of the diet

Food	Not allowed	Allowed
Meat	Preserved or processed meats, bacon, sausage	All other meats
Fish	Smoked fish, shellfish	White fish
Vegetables	Potatoes, onions, corn, eggplant, chilies, bell peppers, tomatoes	All other vegetables, salads, legumes, parsnip and rutebega
Fruit	Citrus fruit e.g. oranges, grapefruit	All other fruit, e.g. apples, bananas, pears
Cereals	Wheat, oats, barley, rye, corn	(Ground) rice, rice flakes & cakes, sago, rice cereals, tapioca, millet, buckwheat
Cooking oils	Corn oil, vegetable oil, peanut oil	Sunflower oil, soy oil, safflower oil, olive oil
Dairy products	Cow's milk, yogurt, butter, eggs, most margarines & cheese	Goat, sheep, and soy milks and products made from them, dairy and trans fat-free margarines
Beverages	Tea, coffee (for adults: all coffee, alcohol), orange and grapefruit juices, tap water	Herbal teas, fresh fruit juices, pure tomato juice (without additives), mineral and distilled water
Miscellaneous	Chocolates, yeast and yeast-extracts, artificial preservatives, colorings and flavorings, monosodium glutamate, all artificial sweeteners	Carob, sea salt, herbs, spices, and small amounts of sugar or honey

After two weeks re-introduce foods in this order: tap water, potatoes, cow's milk, yeast, tea, rye, butter, onions, eggs, steel-cut oats, chocolate, barley, citrus fruits, corn, cow's milk cheese, shellfish, natural cow's milk yogurt, vinegar, wheat, and nuts (and for adults, coffee and wine).

Give only one new food every two days and if there is a reaction, don't try it again for at least a month. Carry on with the list when any symptoms stop. Any diet which is very restricted puts children's health at risk and though it is all right to experiment on your own for a few weeks, any long-term removal of major food groups should only be done under professional guidance, such as a doctor or nutritionist.

hyperactivity & adhd

The symptoms of hyperactivity are all too familiar to many luckless parents and teachers. Hyperactive children are constantly overactive, have poor co-ordination, a short attention span, and little concentration; they are emotionally unstable, prone to violent outbursts, and find it hard to go to bed and often even harder to get to sleep.

In recent years there has been much controversy surrounding the question of hyperactive children, whose problem is called attention deficit hyperactivity disorder, or ADHD. This term does not apply to those who are simply naughty, badly behaved, or difficult. It applies to children who are impossibly disruptive, destructive to themselves and to property, and have learning difficulties.

For years these children were treated exclusively as behaviorally disturbed. Then, in the late 1960s, Dr. Ben Feingold, an allergist working in America, stumbled across a possible chemical cause for hyperactivity while working on a project connected to flea-bite allergies in children. He devised a special diet which excluded a group of chemicals called salicylates, related to the aspirin family and similar to the substances produced by fleas. A number of children who were extremely allergic to flea bites were put on this diet and Feingold was astounded to discover that not only were the children reacting less severely to the flea bites, but their behavior had improved as well.

He then began a major study on hyperactive children who had been institutionalized as they were beyond control. A considerable percentage of the children responded dramatically to the diet, their behavior changing within days. When they were given a doughnut filled with artificially colored and flavored jam, their behavior

deteriorated within hours. Dr Feingold had established that many of the chemicals used as artificial food additives were salicylates, and he suggested that these very chemicals, along with natural salicylates occurring in some foods, were the root of the problem for some children.

chemical offenders

All children with ADHD may be sensitive to some of the chemicals used in processed foods. Among the worst offenders is the yellow coloring, tartrazine (E102), which is widely used in convenience foods, especially in many of the drinks, candies, and cookies aimed directly at the children's market. Many children have been restored to reasonable behavior and sleep by avoiding food additives – some of which can also be the trigger for asthmatic attacks, eczema, urticaria, and other itches and irritations.

Phosphoric acid (E338-341), used in drinks to give them a fresh tingle in the mouth, may be a special problem. Phosphates turn up in other processed foods, including sausages and cooked or processed meats. Phosphoric acid was for a long time believed to be a harmless additive with no known adverse effects. But a German pharmacist, Hertha Hafer, has pointed out that phosphate use in foodstuffs has trebled since the 1960s, and she is firmly convinced that phosphates are a contributing cause for the rising epidemic of hyperactivity among children in many countries.

Hertha's own son Michael was hyperactive, and for a while both Hertha, her husband, and the boy's teachers were delighted with his obvious improvement on doses of Ritalin, the medication now given to millions of "problem children" (see page 210).

After learning of Feingold's work and putting it into practice, however, Hertha became particularly suspicious of phosphoric acid. In her book, *The Hidden Drug*, published in France and Germany, she detailed cases where behavioral problems disappeared once phosphates were withdrawn from the diet. She also suggested a simple kitchen remedy for hyperactivity which she claimed is almost as effective as a tablet of Ritalin – a teaspoon of cider vinegar mixed into a glass of water.

There are other reasons why excess phosphates should be eliminated from children's diets. They can interfere with calcium uptake, leading to poor bone formation and osteoporosis in later life.

Nutritional deficiencies caused by poor diet may be at the root of many cases of hyperactivity. A study in Britain in 1997 indicates that too little zinc may be a cause. The Hyperactive Children's Support Group tested 190 children with ADHD, and found that 183 were deficient in zinc. The research also showed essential fatty acid deficiency: there was marked improvement in children given 2000–3000mg of evening primrose oil a day.

Other vital nutrients are the B-vitamin complex, found in meat and wholegrains; magnesium, found in bananas and dried fruits, cashews, and peanuts; whole wheat flour, brown rice, and green vegetables; and the healthy fats found in oily fish like sardines, mackerel, salmon, and tuna.

the adhd diet

For many hyperactive children, this diet is like turning a switch and going from darkness to light. Some children are just plain badly behaved and need discipline, and others have psychological problems, totally unrelated to food, that lead to their behavioral disorder. No matter what the cause, all children will benefit from the healthier eating patterns you can achieve with this diet.

It is not necessary to follow the plan under medical supervision, although it is easier if you have some help and guidance. You are not removing any entire food groups and you can continue to feed your child on a varied, well-balanced diet. The program is suitable for children over the age of two years whom you suspect of having a behavioral problem and that it might be linked to food chemicals.

1. Keep a diet diary and write down everything your child eats. It is important to keep this diary going even after any improvements have occurred. Keep a column in the diary for general behavior and school progress. If the diet is working, but there is any sudden deterioration in behavior, suspect that one or other of the suspected foods has crept in, either by accident or by cheating.

2. Any fruit or vegetable which is not on the prohibited list of Group 1 (see page 208) is allowed unless you suspect that it causes problems.

3. Be a label reader, rejecting anything that is not 100 percent free of artificial additives. Permitted and not-permitted foods are in the Group 2 lists (see page 209).

4. All children enjoy the occasional sweet treat but you will have to make cakes, cookies, pies, pastries, desserts, and even simple candies at home. Make your own ice cream, too, to avoid the additives in commercially manufactured ones.

5. The best way to guarantee success is to get the whole family following the diet – would you like to watch while everyone else is eating goodies that you are not allowed? The restriction on fresh fruits and the two vegetables can be relaxed after

four to six weeks. Only give one new food in any 48-hour period so you can spot those that might still present a problem.

6. To succeed, the diet must be a 100 percent effort. If an affected child has a mouthful of tartrazine on Sunday, and another on Wednesday, hyperactivity for a week could be the result.

7. Usually, a good response will be obvious within seven to 21 days. In some children behavioral improvements may be noticed within two or three days, in others it might take seven weeks. If your child is one of those sensitive to, or allergic to, these chemicals then you will see a benefit for all your efforts, so persevere.

8. Severely hyperactive children are frequently prescribed behavior-modifying drugs, and you should never make changes without consulting the doctor who is overseeing your child.

group 1

The fruits and vegetables in this list contain natural salicylates, which have been found to be a cause of hyperactivity in children.

They must be omitted in any and all forms – fresh, frozen, canned, dried, as juice, or as an ingredient of prepared foods.

Foods containing natural salicylates

Almonds

Apples

Apricots

Berries: blackberries, raspberries, strawberries, and currants

Cherries

Cucumbers (pickles)

Grapes and raisins or any product made of grapes (wine, wine vinegar, jellies, etc.)

Nectarines

Oranges

(grapefruit, lemon, and lime are permitted)

Peaches

Plums and prunes

Tomatoes and all tomato products

After these foods have been left out of the diet for 4–6 weeks, try them again one at a time for 3 or 4 days. If there is no unfavorable reaction, another item can be added. This procedure is followed until all items in the group are tested and those to which there is no adverse reaction are restored to the diet.

group 2

All foods that contain artificial colors and artificial flavors are prohibited.

The list on the opposite page is a guide for shopping and food preparation. It does not list all foods that contain artificial colors and flavors because it would not be practical to do so. Do not use any foods that contain these substances.

The safest approach is to read food labels carefully and not to buy or use any that contain artificial color and flavors. There is an increasing number of foods available that contain neither.

There are some permitted food items that must be prepared at home to avoid synthetics.

Note: it should be emphasized that this diet is not concerned with food preservatives except for Butylated Hydroxy Toluene (BHT). Occasionally, a child may show an adverse response to BHT.

Foods containing artificial colors and artificial flavors

Food	Not permitted	Permitted
Cereals	All cereals with artificial colors and flavors, all instant-breakfast preparations	Any cereal without artificial colors or flavors, dry or cooked
Bakery Goods	All manufactured cakes, pastries, sweet rolls, doughnuts, etc., pie crusts, frozen baked goods, all commercial breads except egg bread and whole wheat bread, many packaged baking mixes	Any product without artificial color or flavor, but most baked items must be prepared at home

100 percent whole wheat |
Meats	Bologna, salami, hot dogs, sausages, meat loaf, ham, bacon, pork	All other meats
Poultry	All barbecued types, all turkeys with prepared basting called "self-basting," prepared stuffing	All poultry except stuffed
Fish	Frozen fish fillets that are dyed or flavored; fish sticks that are dyed or flavored	All fresh fish
Desserts	Manufactured ice creams, unless the label specifies no synthetic coloring or flavoring; the same applies to sherbet, ices, gelatins, junkets, puddings, and all pudding mixes; all dessert mixes; commercial flavored yogurts.	Homemade ice cream without artificial coloring or flavoring; gelatin desserts, homemade from pure gelatins, with any permitted natural fruit or fruit juices; tapioca; homemade custards and puddings; plain yogurt – fresh fruits or juice may be added
Sweets	All manufactured types, hard or soft	Homemade sweets without almonds
Beverages	Cider, wine, and beer (for adults), diet juices, soft drinks; all instant breakfast drinks; all quick-mix powdered drinks; tea, prepared chocolate milk, coffee	Grapefruit and pineapple juices, pear and guava nectars; homemade lemonade or limeade, made from fresh lemons or limes; milk
Miscellaneous	Any margarine containing artificial additives; colored butter; mustard, cider vinegar, wine vinegar; all mint-flavored items; soy sauce, if flavored or colored; commercial chocolate syrup; barbecue-flavored potato chips; cloves; ketchup; chili sauce

Colored cheeses | All cooking oils and fats; butter icing, not colored or flavored; mustard prepared at home from pure powder and distilled vinegar; honey; preserves, jams, or jellies made from permitted fruits, not artificially colored or flavored; homemade mayonnaise; distilled white vinegar; homemade chocolate syrup

All natural (white) cheeses |
| Sundry Items | All toothpastes; all mouthwashes, cough drops, throat lozenges; antacid tablets, and perfumes | A salt-and-baking soda mixture can be used instead of toothpaste |

diet changes or Ritalin?

Further evidence of the links between food additives and ADHD have became apparent through the work of the criminologist Professor Steven Schoenthaler, at Cal State University, Turlock, California. He conducted studies into the link between food additives and behavior with juvenile delinquents who showed dramatic improvements in behavior within weeks of being given a monitored diet.

Schoenthaler subsequently carried out more studies and concluded that a combination of improved diet and simple multivitamin-mineral supplements could change intelligence and behavior in delinquent young people.

Institutions throughout the country have followed his lead and replaced junk food full of additives with un-processed food, high-fat, and high-sugar items with healthier options, and they have introduced nutritional supplements. The entire New York State public school system has applied Schoenthaler's findings, switching to healthier food and seeing an almost instant improvement in children's learning skills, behavior, and achievement.

The most disturbing feature of ADHD is the current vogue for the prescription of the drug Ritalin. This drug is believed to be taken by around a million children in the US, including 12 percent of boys in the 6–14 age group. In the UK, where nearly 70,000 children are believed to suffer from the most severe form of ADHD, Ritalin was recently approved by the National Institute for Clinical Excellence for use with children suffering from the most severe form of attention disorder.

The clinical advice is that Ritalin should only be used for children who fail to respond to psychotherapy, and the "special precautions" say it must only be used under the supervision of a specialist in behavior disorders. Many people, including concerned parents, suspect that it is routinely prescribed on the insistence of desperate parents, long before other treatments have been explored and without the specialist supervision considered so important.

Children are often on this drug for long periods, side effects are common, and withdrawal is often difficult. Ritalin is a "controlled drug," classified with other highly addictive substances. Before you allow your child to to take this drug for what may be a long time, it is surely worth a few weeks of time and a bit of extra trouble to try the diet suggested here.

eating disorders

Research into eating disorders among children recently found that as many as one in 100 young girls suffers from anorexia nervosa. Figures show the disease is rising among boys, too.

Anorexia nervosa was once a disease of the late teens; therapists are now seeing victims as young as nine and ten. Similar figures are reported from other affluent countries. The researchers also found that those who routinely skipped meals were 18 times more likely to develop anorexia, and even those who simply regularly cut down the amount they ate were five times more likely to develop it at some time.

It is essential for parents to realize that they themselves may have a negative influence on children's attitudes to food. If children see their parents constantly embarking on one diet after another, if they hear them counting calories and checking the fat content on every label, being obsessive about their own weight, or constantly worrying about the rest of the family's, they will receive a powerful message that thin is good and food is bad.

On the other hand, obese children are at considerable risk of becoming obese adults, which is not good for their health either. It is well recognized that some children have a greater tendency to put on weight than others. But the answer for such children can never be a slimming diet: it must always be a combination of healthy eating and exercise.

anorexia nervosa

Anorexia nervosa is a serious eating disorder that has grave long-term health consequences and is frequently a cause of death in young people. It is estimated that between 1 and 2 percent of all schoolgirls suffer with this problem, which is almost exclusively confined to affluent countries. Although the majority of sufferers are girls, up to 10 percent of sufferers are now young boys.

A major factor in the spread of anorexia nervosa is the influence of the media. Advertizing and fashion industries create fashionable, idealized body images, and the multi-million dollar slimming industry pushes diet books, pills, and potions. All this puts pressure on young people to be thin.

Anorexia nervosa is a very complicated illness which inevitably involves social as well as psychological and biological factors, and some new evidence is beginning to show that there is a genetic factor as well. In principle, anorexics are turning their back on sexuality and adolescence, and in girls the cessation of periods frequently precedes the obvious and dramatic weight loss.

the signs of anorexia

Like alcoholics, anorexics become extremely clever at covering up their tracks. Be suspicious if your child starts wearing very baggy clothes, has frequent excuses for not appearing at family meals, or stops going out with friends for hamburgers or a pizza. Parents may sometimes collude unwittingly by accepting their child's concern with food allergies, or a sudden switch to vegetarianism, veganism, or some extreme faddish diet for moral or quasi-religious reasons.

More than half of anorexics become depressed and totally preoccupied with food and its calorie content and with their own body image. Anorexics seem to have fixed on a weight of 98 lb/45kg as their maximum supportable weight, and their lives revolve around staying below this.

Osteoporosis is a major hazard in anorexia. Many young anorexic girls in their late teens and early twenties have bones so thin and weak that they are at serious risk of spinal or hip fractures from the most minor of injuries. The whole metabolic system shuts down in anorexics. The circulatory system suffers, fingers, toes, and lips can be blue-tinged, and hair loss, bad skin, and low blood pressure are all common symptoms.

Although they are obviously emaciated, sufferers become obsessed with the idea that they are fat. This often is the result of peer pressure, parents' over-concern with weight, and also a great fear of growing up. Difficult mother/daughter relationships are also common and there may well be a history of emotional trauma or disturbance before the onset of the illness. Divorce and death of a parent or sibling, are also common triggers.

All forms of treatment are rejected by serious sufferers of anorexia and no amount of persuading will change their own perception of how they look.

treating anorexia nervosa

No parent should attempt to treat anorexia without medical help. The idea of easily getting seriously anorexic children or teenagers to follow a "healthy diet" is ludicrous, just as pandering to the sufferer's eating obsessions is dangerous.

Many parents, especially those in the affluent, higher-income classes from which most cases of anorexia nervosa come, are so anxious about how they will look in the eyes of friends and colleagues if it becomes public knowledge that their child is anorexic, that they delay getting the right care for their child.

Often, the only solution for doctors is to have the patient compulsorily admitted to a psychiatric unit, ideally one that specializes in treatment of the condition. As well as medical treatment to provide massive calorie input, psychotherapy that includes the whole family is essential once the patient's weight has increased to a non-critical level. Anorexics who have effective treatment have a geat chance of survival – 20 years later 95 percent will still be alive – but, left to their own devices and unhelped, 20 percent of sufferers will probably have died.

bulimia nervosa

Bulimia nervosa involves alternate starving and binging. Sufferers can eat huge quantities of food in one sitting, then purge themselves with laxatives or make themselves vomit before returning to their starvation diet. Bulimics are not that easy to spot; they're usually older than anorexics, around the mid-20s being common. They are mostly independent, living away from home, and their normal "diet" is just about socially acceptable. They are seldom emaciated; although sometimes very slim, they may also be overweight.

Bulimia is triggered by the same factors as anorexia: low self-esteem, pressure from ambitious parents, lack of parental affection and attention, and frequently an underlying thread of stress, anxiety, and depression.

helping eating disorders through diet

A main route to helping children and young people with eating disorders is through diet. Anorexics must be encouraged to eat anything that contains calories and nutrients, especially high-zinc foods like shellfish, pumpkin seeds, liver, cheese, beef, and sardines, since zinc stimulates appetite. All foods are acceptable for someone who is very underweight, but it is important to avoid bran and bran-based cereals because they interfere with zinc and iron absorption: anorexics are frequently obsessed with improving bowel function and may use bran as an alternative to laxatives.

The healthiest calories come from complex carbohydrates like whole wheat bread, oats, potatoes, pasta, rice, and beans. But these are very bulky and there is a limit to how much can be eaten at one time. Make sure that these foods contribute at least half the food intake.

Get extra calories from bananas, nuts – as long as they're unsalted or not covered in chocolate – and dried fruits. Raisins, dates, and dried apricots are excellent sources of energy, vitamins, and minerals and also supply useful quantities of fiber. As snacks throughout the day they supply a significant number of calories in comparatively small amounts of food. One of the best sources of healthy calories are seeds; include them in spreads along with nuts. Sunflower and sesame seeds are especially good and are rich in nutrients: tahini, a spread made from crushed sesame, and peanut butter provide a large number of calories with little bulk.

the value of frequent snacking

Try to encourage eating every two hours, starting at breakfast and finishing with a bedtime snack. Dips like guacamole, made from avocado and olive oil, or hummus, made with chickpeas and tahini, eaten with whole wheat pita bread, make an excellent between-meals snack and, like all the best foods, provide a high proportion of nutrients along with their calories.

Finally, try this recipe. Make it up first thing in the morning, encourage your child to have a glass before breakfast, keep the rest in the refrigerator and make sure it's all gone by bedtime. Put 2½ cups/600ml whole milk, one certified salmonella-free raw egg, one banana, 2 teaspoons each of molasses, honey, tahini, wheatgerm, and brewer's yeast powder, and four dried apricots into a blender. Whisk the ingredients together, pour into a pitcher and keep in the refrigerator. (The recipe could be made in a bowl, using a hand blender.)

why zinc is important

Brains need zinc. Confusion, depression, including the "baby blues" (post-partum depression), even schizophrenia have been linked with low zinc levels. Since both appetite and taste depend on zinc, lack of the mineral can be one cause of anorexia nervosa. There are well-documented cases of anorexics making spectacular recoveries when given extra zinc. High stress levels, growth, and hormonal turmoil make teenagers vulnerable to zinc deficiency, especially if they're dieting.

If your child is anorexic, it's well worth checking zinc levels, and there's a simple way to do it. Buy from a chemist a bottle of distilled or de-ionized water and a pack of zinc capsules containing 50mg elemental zinc. Open one up and stir the contents into 1 cup/225ml of the distilled water. To those well supplied with zinc, the water will have a strong metallic taste. If it tastes like water, they're dangerously low.

The supplemental dose is also 50mg of elemental zinc a day, taken with food or at least a fruit juice, until the sense of taste returns. Repeat the test dose to check. The dose can be increased up to three times a day, but no higher. It should be reduced as soon as possible.

If appetite does return, a good zinc-rich diet will be life-saving. Good sources of zinc include liver, red meat, turkey, crabmeat, sardines, eggs, kidney beans, chickpeas and wholegrain bread.

resources

* *

American Community Garden Network
www.communitygarden.org
100 N 20th St., 5th Floor
Philadelphia, PA 19103-1495
tel: 215-988-8785
Non-profit organization dedicated to supporting
community gardens in urban and rural areas.

AMS Farmers' Markets
www.ams.usda.gov/directmarketing
A national directory of farmers' markets.

Canadian Organics Advisory Board
www.coab.ca
206 Seventh Avenue SW, Suite 506
Calgary, AB, Canada T2P 0W7
tel: 403-262-4640
A non-profit organization committed to organic
standards and certification.

Canada's Organic Community
www.inforganics.com
A non-profit organization dedicated to bringing
together people with interests in organics.

Center for Food Safety
www.centerforfoodsafety.org
666 Pennsylvania Ave SE, Suite 302
Washington, DC 20003
tel: 202-547-9359

Dietitians of Canada
www.dietitians.ca
480 University Avenue, Suite 604
Toronto, ON, Canada M5G 1V2
tel: 416-596-0857
Canadian association promoting health through
food and nutrition.

Eating Disorders Awareness and Prevention, Inc.
www.edap.org
603 Stewart Street, Suite 803
Seattle, WA 98101

tel: 206-382-3587
Non-profit organization devoted to the
awareness and prevention of eating disorders.

Farm Verified Organic
www.textcity.com/farm
5449 45th Street SE
Medina, ND 58467
tel: 701-486-3578
International organic certification organization.

Feingold Association
www.feingold.org
127 East Main Street, Suite 106
Riverhead, NY 11901
tel: 631-369-9340
Research organization on the connection
between ADHD and children's diets.

Friends of the Earth (FOE)
www.foe.org/safefood
1025 Vermont Ave NW
Washington, DC 20005-6303
tel: 202-783-7400
Association of organizations dedicated
to protecting the environment.

Juvenile Diabetes Foundation of Canada
www.jdfc.ca
7100 Woodbine Avenue, Suite 311
Markham, ON, Canada L3R 5J2
tel: 905-944-8700
Charitable organization providing awareness,
education, and support to children with diabetes.

La Leche League International
www.lalecheleague.org
PO Box 4079
Schaumburg, IL 60173
tel: 847-519-7730
Non-profit organization dedicated to providing
education, support, and encouragement to
women who want to breast-feed.

Independent Organic Inspectors Association
www.ioia.net
PO Box 6
Broadus, MT 59317
tel: 406-436-2031
Non-profit organization of trained, qualified farm inspectors dedicated to verification of organic products.

Mothers and Others for a Livable Planet
www.igc.apc.org/mothers
40 West 20th Street
New York, NY 10011-4211
tel: 212-24-0010
Organization dedicated to market choices for a safer, healthier environment.

National Eating Disorder Information Center
www.nedic.on.ca
CW1-211, 200 Elizabeth Street
Toronto, ON, Canada M5G 2C4
tel: 416-340-4156
Non-profit origanization providing information on eating disorders and weight problems.

National Institues of Diabetes and Digestive and Kidney Diseases
www.niddk.nih.gov
US National Institutes of Health information on helping your overweight child.

National Organic Directory Community Alliance with Family Farmers (CAFF)
www.caff.org
PO Box 363
Davis, CA 95617-9900
tel: 530-756-8518
An annual directory that provides information on farmers, wholesalers, manufacturers/processors, and retailers, certification groups, and farm suppliers.

Organic Kitchen
www.organickitchen.com
Websites with links focusing on organic food products, research, and marketing.

Organic Trade Association
www.ota.com
A resource directory with listings for over 530 certified organic farms in North America.

Rodale Institute
www.rodaleinstitute.org
611 Siegfrieddale Road
Kutztown, PA 19530
tel: 800-823-6285
Worldwide organization devoted to achieving a regenerative food system.

Toronto Vegetarian Association
www.veg.on.ca
2300 Yonge St., Suite 1101
PO Box 2307
Toronto, ON, Canada M4P 1E4
tel: 416-544-9800
Organization devoted to helping people to adopt and maintain a healthful, vegetarian lifestyle.

Union of Concerned Scientists
www.ucsusa.org
2 Brattle Square
Cambridge, MA 02238-9105
tel: 617-547-5552
Organization of scientists dedicated to achieving a healthful, clean, secure environment.

USDA for Kids
www.usda.gov/news/usdakids
A nutrition website for children.

USDA National Organic Program
www.ams.usda.gov/nop
US standards for organic agricultural production.

Vegetarian Baby and Child
www.vegetarianbaby.com
PO Box 519
Tuolumne, CA 95379
Educates families about the diets of vegetarian and vegan children.

books to read

FOOD AND NUTRITION BOOKS:

The Catalog of Healthy Food
John Tepper Marlin, Ph.D.
BANTAM BOOKS, New York 1990

A Consumer Dictionary of
Food Additives
Ruth Winter
CROWN PUBLISHERS, 1989

Food Your Miracle Medicine
Jean Carper
SIMON & SCHUSTER, 1993

The Natural Baby Food Cookbook
Margaret Elizabeth Kenda
& Phyllis S. Williams
AVON BOOKS, 1982

Nutritional Medicine: a Comprehensive Guide
to Nutrition in Medicine
Dr Stephen Davies and Dr Alan Stewart
PAN BOOKS, 1987
Includes useful sections on individual nutrients,
their function, food sources of them and
deficiency symptoms.

Nature's Kitchen: The Complete
Guide to the New American Diet
Fred Rohe
STOREY COMMUNICATIONS, 1986

Organic Baby and Toddler Cookbook
Lizzie Vann
DK PUBLISHING, Inc., New York, 2001

Organic Cookbook
Renée Elliott & Eric Treuille
DK Publishing, Inc., New York, 2001

Poisoning Our Children:
Surviving in a Toxic World
Nancy Sokol Green
THE NOBLE PRESS, 1991

Prevention's Healthy Cookbook
Rodale & Staff
RODEL PRESS, 2000

GARDENING BOOKS:

The Organic Garden Book
Geoff Hamilton
DORLING KINDERSLEY, 1999

Square Foot Gardening
Mel Bartholomew
RODEL PRESS, 1981

index

Page numbers in **bold** indicate superfood main entries.
Page numbers in *italics* indicate recipes and quick food ideas.

A
additives 22, 68, 206
ADHD exclusion diet 207-9
ADHD & hyperactivity 206-10
allergies & intolerances, food 44, 61, 202-5
almonds **45**, *46*
    banana & almond muffins *163*
    chickpea veggie burgers *182*
    veggie burgers with spinach cheese topping *182*
amaranth **51**
ancient grains **51**
anorexia nervosa 211-12, 213
antioxidants & vitamins 20-1, 75, 77
apples **34**, 93, 100, 105
    apple & apricot purée *124*
    baked apples *199*
    beet & apple soup *132*
        blackberry & apple crumble *189*
    brown rice with apple purée *48, 173*
    coleslaw *198*
    dark fruit drink *194*
    Granny Smith's Welsh rarebit *155, 198*
    kiwi surprise *192*
    moist apple bread *159*
    nutty apple juice *194*
    pear power *194*
    red cabbage with apple & chestnuts *181*
    stewed apple with mascarpone *191*
    whole wheat pancakes with apple purée *47*
apricot purée, apple & *124*
apricot scones *159*
apricots *38*, **38**
artificial sweeteners 68

asparagus *27*, **27**
aspartame 68
avocado dip *149*
avocado sauce, pasta with *175*
avocados *33*, **33**, 80, 112

B
b plus *195*
babies, breast-feeding & baby meals 78-83
bacon **53**
    baked eggs & bacon *125*
    mushrooms on toast with crumbly cheese *153, 198*
    potato cakes with broiled bacon *171*
    red cabbage with apple & chestnuts *181*
baked apples *199*
baked eggs & bacon *125*
baked potatoes *199*
baked Savoy cabbage soup with melted cheese *132*
balanced diet *see* nutrition & healthy eating
bananas **38**, 89
    banana & almond muffins *163*
    banana & walnut bread *163*
    banana cereal *120*
    banana-to-go *124*
    lime-e-shake *124*
    mighty muesli munchies *158*
    milk drink for children with eating disorders *213*
    nutty apple juice *194*
bannocks *127*
barley **50**
barley bannocks *127*
basil **64**
bay leaves **65**
beans
    dried *see* dried & canned beans
    green *see* green beans
beef **52**
    beefburgers as danger foods 52, 67
    classic Bolognese sauce *177*

radar burgers *184*
beets **30**
beet & apple soup *132*
berries **36-7**
    berry delight *192*
    blackberry & apple crumble *189*
    blueberry muffins *162*
    summer pudding *188*
black bean chili *168*
blackberries **36**
blackberry & apple crumble *189*
blood sugar levels 14
blueberries **36**
blueberry muffins *162*
Bolognese sauce, classic *177*
Brazil nuts **45**
bread 89, 93, *198*
    baked Savoy cabbage soup with melted cheese *132*
    bread & cheese bake *198*
    bread & tomato salad *147*
    eggy triangles *61*
    hot pancetta savories *154*
    oven-baked beans *196*
    ploughman's lunch (or supper) *59, 198*
    quick spinach snack *154*
    sandwich fillings *47, 61, 156*
    summer pudding *188*
    tomato & cheese bread pudding *143*
    vegetable nests with crunchy cheese topping *141*
    see also burgers; pita bread; pizzas; toast
breads, homemade
    banana & walnut *163*
    bread with oatmeal *49*
    cheese pretzels *157*
    green tea *161*
    hot cross buns *161*
    moist apple *159*
    quick & easy whole wheat *150*
breakfast cereals 69
breast-feeding 78-9
broccoli **27**, 76, 80
    broccoli & anchovy pasta *175*

broccoli *continued*
  broccoli, green bean & sweet
    potato purée *136*
  broccoli with potatoes *146*
  broccoli with spinach *180*
  broccoli stir-fried with ginger &
    garlic *146*
  cauliflower & broccoli cheese
    171
broth, high-protein tofu *131*
brown rice **48**, 76
  recipes using *see* rice
bubble & squeak *174*
buckwheat **50**, 89
buckwheat crêpes *148*
bulgur wheat **47**
  tabbouleh *47*
  veggie burgers with spinach
    cheese topping *182*
bulimia nervosa 212, 213
buns, hot cross *161*
burgers
  bean *184*
  chicken in a wrap *178*
  chickpea veggie *182*
  as danger foods 52, 67
  freezing 119
  nut *183*
  onion-&-squeak *184*
  radar *184*
  rice *183*
  veggie, with spinach cheese
    topping *182*
butter 16-17, **62**
butters
  mixed-nut *46*
  peanut *see* peanuts & peanut
    butter

C
cabbage 26, **26**
  baked Savoy cabbage soup with
    melted cheese *132*
  bubble & squeak *174*
  colcannon *141*
  coleslaw *198*
  red cabbage with apple &
    chestnuts *181*
caffeine 66
cakes 69

calcium 19
calorie content, fats 17
candy 68
canned beans *see* dried & canned
  beans
carbohydrates 13-14
carrots **28**, 80, 105
  bean burgers *184*
  carrot cake *162*
  coleslaw *198*
  crudités *30*
  high-protein tofu broth *131*
  kiwi surprise *192*
  poached chicken *166*
  stuffed celery sticks *155*
  tomatoes plus *194*
  veggie burgers with spinach
    cheese topping *182*
cashew nuts **46**
cauliflower **27**, 84
cauliflower & broccoli cheese *171*
celeriac **32**
  creamy celery soup *131*
  mashed potatoes with celeriac
    180
celery **32**
  b plus *195*
  chickpea veggie burgers *182*
  creamy celery soup *131*
  stuffed celery sticks *155*
  tomatoes plus *194*
cheese **59**, 113, *198*
  baked potatoes *199*
  baked Savoy cabbage soup with
    melted cheese *132*
  bread & cheese bake *198*
  cauliflower & broccoli cheese
    171
  cheese pretzels *157*
  eggs & spinach mornay *198*
  Granny Smith's Welsh rarebit
    155, *198*
  Greek salad *59*
  mushrooms on toast with
    crumbly cheese *153*, *198*
  oven-baked beans *196*
  pizza baguettes *154*
  pizza-style bread *198*
  ploughman's lunch (or supper)
    59, *198*

rice croquettes *48*, *199*
savory egg *153*
spinach soufflé *152*
stewed apple with mascarpone
  191
tomato & cheese bread pudding
  143
vegetable nests with crunchy
  cheese topping *141*
veggie burgers with spinach
  cheese topping *182*
see also cottage cheese; cream
  cheese; mozzarella cheese
cherries **37**
chestnuts **45**
chestnuts, red cabbage with apple
  & *181*
chicken **54**, 89, 100
  chicken salad with honey &
    chili *138*
  chicken in a wrap *178*
  marinated broiled *138*
  poached *166*
  roast, puréed with vegetables
    167
  sandwich fillings *156*
chickpeas **43**
  chickpea veggie burgers *182*
  vegetable couscous *172*
  vegetable curry with dal *181*
  see also hummus
chicory **31**
chili, black bean *168*
chili peppers **65**
chives **29**, **65**
chocolate 68
chocolate sauce, fruit dipped in
  186
cholesterol 17
cilantro **65**
cinnamon **65**
citrus fruits **35**, 76
classic Bolognese sauce *177*
clementines **35**
cloves **65**
coconut crush *192*
coffee 66
colcannon *141*
coleslaw *198*
cooked cereal 97

breakfast 69
banana *120*
serving suggestions *49, 122*
cookies 69
cooking 7
food & kitchen hygiene
114-15
time-saving tips 119
copper 19
coriander **65**
corn 49, **49**
popcorn 49, *49*
smoked mackerel quiche *140*
tuna & corn salad *49, 198*
corn oil 16-17, **63**
costs, food 8-9
cottage cheese **59**, *199*
b plus *195*
banana & walnut bread *163*
fruit with *59, 199*
Greek salad variation *199*
salad *59*
smoky dip *149*
spinach soufflé *152*
stuffed celery sticks *155*
vegetable samosas *172*
couscous **47**
couscous, vegetable *172*
cow's milk **58**, **59**
cracked wheat *see* bulgur wheat
cranberries **37**
cream **63**
cream cheese
cream-cheese dip *149*
stuffed celery sticks *155*
vegetable samosas *172*
cream of smoked haddock &
potato soup *134*
creamy celery soup *131*
creamy fruit tart *186*
creamy yogurt with nuts & honey
123
crêpes *see* pancakes
croquettes, rice *48*, 199
crudités *30*
crumbles *46, 189*
cucumber & yogurt salad *60*
cumin **65**
currants **41**
curry, vegetable, with dal *181*

D
dairy products **58-60**
allergies 204
see also by name eg yogurt
dal, vegetable curry with *181*
danger foods 6-7, 66-9
babies 81
pre-school children 88, 89
pre-teens 97
pregnancy 74
school children under nine
92, 93
teenagers 101
toddlers 85
vegetarian children 105
when breast-feeding 79
dark fruit drink *194*
dates **41**, 97
mighty muesli munchies *158*
diet *see* eating plans; nutrition &
healthy eating
dips, four dips *149*
disorders *see* food-related
disorders
dried & canned beans **42**
baked beans on toast *42, 196*
bean burgers *184*
beans 'n' onions *196*
black bean chili *168*
Indian kidney beans *185*
minestrone *128*
minestrone with pesto *130*
oven-baked beans *196*
Sophie's Indonesian vegetable
stew *178*
tuna & bean salad *146*
tuna & beans *42, 196*
vegetable curry with dal *181*
dried fruit **41**, 93
fruitfast *124*
drinks *124, 192-5*
cranberry juice *37*
fruit drink with yogurt *60*
fruit juices, diluting 22, 67
lemonade 195
orange juice 35
soft drinks, (carbonated)
commercially produced
22, 66, 67
duck **55**

E
eating disorders 211-13
eating healthily *see* nutrition &
healthy eating
eating plans
ADHD exclusion diet 207-9
allergies exclusion diet 205
babies 78-83
eating disorders 213
pre-conception fitness for men
75
pre-school children 88-91
pre-teens 96-9
pregnancy 74-7
school children under 9 92-5
teenagers 100-3
toddlers 84-7
vegetarian children 104-7
eggs **61**, 93, 97, 115, *198*
allergies 61, 204
baked eggs & bacon *125*
baked potatoes *199*
bread & cheese bake *198*
egg mayonnaise *61*
eggs & spinach mornay *198*
eggy triangles *61*
flavored scrambled eggs *61*
French toast *126*
milk drink for children with
eating disorders *213*
old-fashioned kedgeree *140*
poached egg & tomato *126*
prune purée *191*
rosti-topped fish pie *167*
savory egg *153*
scrambled egg with tomatoes &
mushrooms *125*
tuna & bean salad *146*
tuna-eggs mayonnaise *196*
see also individual dishes
normally made with eggs eg
pancakes
English lemonade *195*
equipment, kitchen 110-11
essential fatty acids 16-17, 23,
207
exclusion diets
ADHD 207-9
allergies 205
exotic fruit **40**

F

fats & oils 16-17, **62-3**, 112
feeding guidelines 72, 118
fennel with lemon & mixed herbs 145
fish **56-7**, 76, 80, 93, 97
  allergies 204
  fish cakes *139*, *153*
  fish soup with rouille, croûtons *135*
  old-fashioned kedgeree *140*
  real fish sticks *166*
  rosti-topped fish pie *167*
  sandwich fillings *156*
  smoked mackerel quiche *140*
  smoky dip *149*
  trout or mackerel rolled in oats *49*
  see also salmon; smoked haddock; tuna
five-grain kruska *123*
flavored scrambled eggs *61*
flour 13-14, **47**
folic acid 21
ffood costs 8-9
food hygiene 114-15
food labeling & slogans 6-7
food-related disorders 201
  allergies & intolerances 44, 61, 202-5
  eating disorders 211-13
  hyperactivity & ADHD 206-10
four dips *149*
French toast *126*
fruit **34-41**, 112
  with cottage cheese 59, *199*
  creamy fruit tart *186*
  fruit dipped in chocolate sauce *186*
  fruit drink with yogurt *60*
  fruitfast *124*
  muesli *120*
  pancakes *190*, *199*
  really fruity yogurt *123*
  summer pudding *188*
  upside-down pudding *188*
  see also by name eg apples

G

gadgets & equipment, kitchen 110-111
garlic **29**, **64**, 112, 119
garlic purée 29

ginger **65**
ginger fruit pudding *189*
glucose 14
gluten allergy 204
goat milk, cheeses & yogurt **58**, **59**, 60
golden raisins **41**
grains **47-51**, 112
  five-grain kruska *123*
  multi-grain pancakes *126*
  see also by name eg rice
Granny Smith's Welsh rarebit *155*, *198*
grapefruit 35
grapes **41**, 89
Greek salads 59, *199*
Greek yogurt *see* yogurt & Greek yogurt
green beans **30**, 105
  broccoli, green bean & sweet potato purée *136*
green peppers *see* sweet bell peppers
green tea bread *161*
guavas *40*, **40**

H

haddock
  haddock moussaka *164*
  and see smoked haddock
ham & mushroom sauce *177*
hazelnut oil **63**
hazelnuts **46**
healthy eating *see* nutrition & healthy eating
herbed kofta kebabs *169*
herbs **64-5**, 112
herring 76
high-protein tofu broth *131*
hot cross buns *161*
hot pancetta savories *154*
hummus 47, *156*
hygiene, kitchen & food 114-15
hyperactivity & ADHD 206-10

I J

ice cream 69
iced lollies, pineapple *39*
Indian kidney beans *185*
insulin 14
intolerances & allergies, food 44,

61, 202-5
iodine 19
Irish stew *168*
iron 19
juice *see* drinks

K

kamut 51
kebabs, herbed kofta *169*
kedgeree, old-fashioned *140*
ketchup, tomato 33
kitchen equipment 110-11
kitchen hygiene 114-15
kiwi surprise *192*
kiwifruit *39*, **39**, 84
kofta kebabs, herbed *169*

L

labeling & slogans, food 6-7
lamb **53**
  black bean chili *168*
  herbed kofta kebabs *169*
  Irish stew *168*
leeks **29**
  baked *29*
  colcannon *141*
  fish soup with rouille & croûtons *135*
  high-protein tofu broth *131*
  leek & watercress soup *131*
  poached chicken *166*
legumes **42-3**
  see also by name eg chickpeas
lemonade *195*
lemons **35**
lentils **43**, 97
lettuce 105
lettuces **31**
lime-e-shake *124*

M

magnesium 18
mandarins **35**
manganese 19
mangoes *40*, **40**
  jungle juice *194*
  tropical delight *195*
marinated grilled chicken *138*
mascarpone, stewed apple with *191*
meal plans *see* eating plans

meat **52-3**, 115
  see also types of meat by name
      eg lamb
melon **34**
men, pre-conception fitness 75
menu plans *see* eating plans
microwaves 115
mighty muesli munchies *158*
milk **58**
  allergies 204
  milk-based drinks *124, 192,
      194, 213*
millet **48**, 84
millet pilaf *48*
minerals 18-19, 75, 77
minestrone soups *128-30*
mint **65**
moist apple bread *159*
monounsaturated fats 16
moussaka, haddock *164*
mozzarella cheese
  hot pancetta savories *154*
  Italian tricolore salad *33*
  mozzarella, tomato, & parmesan
      sauce *176*
  Oliver's pizza *185*
muesli *120*
muesli munchies, mighty *158*
muffins *162, 163*
multi-grain pancakes *126*
mushrooms
  ham & mushroom sauce *177*
  mushrooms on toast with
      crumbly cheese *153, 198*
  scrambled egg with tomatoes &
      mushrooms *125*
  veggie burgers with spinach
      cheese topping *182*

N
nectarines **38**
nutmeg **65**
NutraSweet 68
nutrition & healthy eating
  costs 8-9
  feeding guidelines 72, 118
  food & kitchen hygiene 114-15
  foods to avoid *see* danger foods
  nutrients *see* by name eg protein
  organic foods 22-3, 58, 78-9, 201

plate for life 12-13
  see also eating plans
nuts **44-6**
  allergies 44, 204
  blackberry & apple crumble *189*
  carrot cake *162*
  creamy yogurt with nuts &
      honey *123*
  green tea bread *161*
  mixed-nut butters *46*
  moist apple bread *159*
  multi-grain pancakes *126*
  nut burgers *183*
  red cabbage with apple &
      chestnuts *181*
  in salads *46*
  shortbread trees *162*
  see also almonds
nutty apple juice *194*

O
oats & oatmeal 49, **49**, 93, 100
  oatcakes *158*
  oatmeal bannocks *127*
  see also cooked cereal
oatcakes *158*
oils & fats 16-17, **62-3**, 112
oily fish 16, 17, **57**, 76, 93
old-fashioned kedgeree *140*
olive oil 16-17, **63**, 119
Oliver's pizza *185*
omega-3 & omega-6 fatty acids
  16-17
omelettes
  potato *198-9*
  south of France *169*
  Spanish *145, 198*
onions **29**
  beans 'n' onions *196*
  onion-&-squeak burgers *184*
  roasted onions *29*
  sausage supper *199*
  Spanish omelette *145, 198*
oranges **35**, 97
  fruit drink with yogurt *60*
  lime-e-shake *124*
oregano **64**
organic foods 22-3, 58, 78-9, 201
oven-baked beans *196*
overnight cereal *122*

P
pancakes *47, 190, 199*
  bannocks *127*
  buckwheat crêpes *148*
  multi-grain pancakes *126*
pancetta savories, hot *154*
papayas **40**
parsley **64**, 119
passionfruit, jungle juice *194*
pasta **47**, 112, 119, *199*
  pasta & cherry tomatoes *33*
  pasta salad with tuna *147*
  sauces for 175-7
peaches **38**, 119
peanuts & peanut butter **45**
  nutty apple juice *194*
  sandwich fillings *156*
pears
  dark fruit drink *194*
  pear power *194*
peas, split (dried) *see* split peas
peppers *see* chili peppers; sweet
  bell peppers
pesto, minestrone with *130*
pesto & tomato tarts *143*
pilafs *48, 51*
pine nuts **46**
pineapples **39**
  ice pops *39*
  pear power *194*
  sorbet *39*
  tropical delight *195*
pistachio nuts **45**
pisto *144*
pita bread
  fillings for *55, 156*
  pita pizzas *47*
  pita plus *149*
pizzas
  Oliver's pizza *185*
  pita pizzas *47*
  pizza baguettes *154*
  pizza-style bread *198*
plate for life 12-13
ploughman's lunch (or supper)
  59, 198
poached chicken *166*
poached egg & tomato *126*
polenta 49
polyunsaturated fats 16

popcorn 49, *49*
pork **53**
potassium 19
potatoes *28*, **28**, 89, 112
　baked potatoes *199*
　bean burgers *184*
　broccoli with potatoes *146*
　bubble & squeak *174*
　colcannon *141*
　cream of smoked haddock & potato soup *134*
　creamy celery soup *131*
　fish cakes *153*
　fishy feast *139*
　Irish stew *168*
　leek & watercress soup *131*
　mashed potato & celeriac *180*
　onion-&-squeak burgers *184*
　poached chicken *166*
　potato cakes with broiled bacon *171*
　potato chips *69*
　potato omelette *198-9*
　potatoes Juventus *28*
　pumpkin soup *133*
　root vegetable & potato purée *136*
　rosti-topped fish pie *167*
　salmon fish cakes *139*
　sausage supper *199*
　Spanish omelette *145*, *198*
　tuna & potato salad *196*
　tuna mash *152*
　vegetable samosas *172*
poultry **54-5**, 115
　pita bread filling *55*
　see also by name eg chicken
pre-conception fitness plan for men 75
pre-school children, eating plan 88-91
pre-teens, eating plan 96-9
pregnancy, eating plan 74-7
processed fish 56
protein 15-16
prunes **41**
　dark fruit drink *194*
　prune purée *191*
　rabbit with prunes *166*
pumpkin **30**

pumpkin seeds **46**
pumpkin soup *133*
pyridoxine 21

Q
quiche, smoked mackerel *140*
quick & easy whole wheat bread *150*
quick spinach snack *154*
quinoa *51*, **51**
　peppers stuffed with *144*

R
rabbit **53**
rabbit with prunes *166*
radar burgers *184*
radishes 105
raisins **41**
rarebit, Granny Smith's Welsh *155*, *198*
raspberries **36**
raw tomato & red pepper sauce *176*
raw tomato sauce *176*
ready-to-eat refrigerated foods, food safety 115
real fish sticks *166*
real rice pudding *191*
red cabbage with apple & chestnuts *181*
red currants **37**
red peppers *see* sweet bell peppers
refrigerator & freezer
　food safety 115
　home freezing 119
　suggested contents 113
reheating food 115
riboflavin 21
rice **48**, *199*
　brown rice with apple purée *48*, *173*
　brown rice four ways *173*
　croquettes *48*
　minestrone with rice & tomatoes *130*
　old-fashioned kedgeree *140*
　quick food ideas with cooked rice *48*
　real rice pudding *191*
　rice burgers *183*
　rice croquettes *199*

rice water **48**
Sophie's Indonesian vegetable stew *178*
split pea & rice soup *134*
stir-fries with cooked rice *199*
veggie burgers with spinach cheese topping *182*
Ritalin 210
roast chicken puréed with vegetables *167*
roasted vegetables *174*
rolled oats **49**
root vegetable & potato purée *136*
rosemary **64**
rosti-topped fish pie *167*
rye **50**

S
safflower oil 16-17, **63**
sage **64**
salads **31-3**, 113
　bread & tomato *147*
　brown rice four ways *173*
　chicken, with honey & chili *138*
　coleslaw *198*
　cottage cheese *59*
　cucumber & yogurt *60*
　Greek *59*, *199*
　Italian tricolore *33*
　nuts in *46*
　pasta, with tuna *147*
　tabbouleh *47*
　tuna & bean *146*
　tuna & potato *196*
　tuna & corn *49*, *198*
　tuna-eggs mayonnaise *196*
　see also individual salad vegetables by name eg tomatoes
salmon 84, 100
　fish cakes *153*
　salmon fish cakes *139*
　salmon surprise *152*
samosas, vegetable *172*
sandwich fillings *47*, *61*, *156*
　for pita bread *55*, *149*, *156*
sardines 93
satsumas **35**
saturated fats 16-17
sausage supper *199*
savory egg *153*

school children, eating plans
    pre-teens 96-9
    teenagers 100-3
    under 9s 92-5
scones, apricot 159
seeds 44, 46
allergies 204
    cheese pretzels 157
    vegetable samosas 172
    see also sunflower seeds
selenium 18
semolina 47
sesame seeds 46, 100
sesame smoothie 195
shallots 29
sheep milk cheeses & yogurt 59, 60
shellfish 56, 57, 76
    allergies 204
shortbread trees 162
shrimp & vegetable stir-fry, Zoë's 164
shrimp 76
slogans & labeling, food 6-7
smoked haddock
    cream of smoked haddock & potato soup 134
    fishy feast 139
smoked mackerel quiche 140
smoky dip 149
soft drinks, commercially produced 22, 66, 67
Sophie's Indonesian vegetable stew 178
sorbet, pineapple 39
soufflé, spinach 152
soups 26, 27, 128-35
    chicken 54
south of France omelette 169
soy beans & soy bean products 43
    see also tofu
soy milk 58
    coconut crush 192
Spanish omelette 145, 198
spelt 51
spices 65, 112
spinach 29, 80
    broccoli with spinach 180
    eggs & spinach mornay 198

quick spinach snack 154
spinach soufflé 152
veggie burgers with spinach cheese topping 182
split peas 43
    chickpea veggie burgers 182
    split pea & rice soup 134
sprouted wheat 47, 47
squash see pumpkin
stewed apple with mascarpone 191
stews 168, 178
stir-fries 146, 164, 199
pantry, suggested contents 112
storing food safely 115
strawberries 36
stuffed celery sticks 155
sugar 67
    blood sugar levels 14
summer pudding 188
sun-dried tomatoes 33
sunflower oil 16-17, 63
sunflower seeds 46, 100
    apricot scones 159
    chickpea veggie burgers 182
    quick & easy whole wheat bread 150
supplements, vitamin 21, 104
sweet bell peppers 29
    Indian kidney beans 185
    peppers stuffed with quinoa 144
    raw tomato & red pepper sauce 176
    smoky dip 149
    Spanish omelette 145, 198
sweet potatoes 28
    broccoli, green bean, & sweet potato purée 136
sweeteners, artificial 68

T

tabbouleh 47
tart, creamy fruit 186
tarts, pesto & tomato 143
tea 66
teenagers, eating plan 100-3
thiamin 21
thyme 64

time-saving cooking tips 119
toast
    baked beans on toast 42, 196
    beans 'n' onions 196
    French toast 126
    Granny Smith's Welsh rarebit 155, 198
    mushrooms on toast with crumbly cheese 153, 198
toddlers, eating plan 84-7
tofu
    high-protein tofu broth 131
    Sophie's Indonesian vegetable stew 178
tomatoes 33, 105, 119
    b plus 195
    bread & tomato salad 147
    flavored scrambled eggs 61
    Italian tricolore salad 33
    minestrone with rice & tomatoes 130
    mozzarella, tomato & parmesan sauce 176
    pasta & cherry tomatoes 33
    pesto & tomato tarts 143
    poached egg & tomato 126
    raw tomato & red pepper sauce 176
    raw tomato sauce 176
    scrambled egg with tomatoes & mushrooms 125
    south of France omelette 169
    tomato & anchovy sauce 177
    tomato & cheese pudding 143
    tomato & yogurt dip 149
    tomatoes plus 194
    tuna & bean salad 146
    see also individual dishes normally made with tomatoes eg pizza
tortillas, chicken in a wrap 178
trans-fats 17
treats 66
tropical delight 195
tuna
    pasta salad with tuna 147
    pita plus 149
    tuna & bean salad 146
    tuna & beans 42, 196

tuna *continued*
  tuna & potato salad *196*
  tuna & corn salad *49, 198*
  tuna-eggs mayonnaise *196*
  tuna mashed potatoes *152*
turkey **55**
turnips **27**, 80

UV

upside-down pudding *188*
utensils, kitchen 110-11
vegetable oils 16-17, **63**
vegetables **26-30**, 112, 113
  colcannon *141*
  minestrone with pesto *130*
  pisto *144*
  roast chicken puréed with *167*
  roasted *174*
  root vegetable & potato purée *136*
  Sophie's Indonesian vegetable stew *178*
  stir-fries with cooked rice *199*
  vegetable couscous *172*
  vegetable curry with dal *181*
  vegetable nests with crunchy

cheese topping *141*
vegetable samosas *172*
veggie burgers *see* burgers
Zoë's shrimp & vegetable stir-fry *164*
see also by name eg cabbage
vegetarian children, eating plan 104-7
venison **53**
vitamins & antioxidants 20-1, 75, 77, 104

W

walnut bread, banana & *163*
walnut oil 17, **63**
walnuts **45**
watercress *32*, **32**, 100
  leek & watercress soup *131*
  pita plus *149*
  stuffed celery sticks *155*
watermelon 34
wheat **47**
  see also individual dishes normally made with wheat eg breads
wheatgerm **47**

white fish **57**, 80
white rice **48**
whole wheat flour **47**
wild berries 37

YZ

yellow bell peppers *see* sweet bell peppers
yogurt & Greek yogurt **60**, 63, 68, 76, 84
  cream-cheese dip *149*
  creamy yogurt with nuts & honey *123*
  fruit with, quick food ideas *38, 40, 60, 199*
  really fruity yogurt *123*
  tomato & yogurt dip *149*
  yogurt-based drinks *124, 192, 194, 195*
  yogurt and cucumber salad *60*
zinc 18, 75, 207, 213
Zoë's shrimp & vegetable stir-fry *164*

acknowledgments & credits

The authors would like to thank Corinne Roberts for her enthusiasm and encouragement; Janice Anderson for her patient and indefatigable editing; art editor Glenda Fisher, who transformed the book into a work of art; and Fiona Lindsay of Limelight Management, our delightful, efficient literary agent.

They would also like to thank Victoria Heath for recipes tested at her child-friendly Cooking School; Mia Perren for original recipes and for recipe-testing; Aldo Zilli for Cream of Smoked Haddock & Potato Soup from *Zilli Fish* (Metro Publishing); Emily Sharman, pupil of a Cookie Crumbles' cooking class for Chicken Salad with Honey & Chili; and Lizzie Vann of Organix for Banana Cereal. Spinach & Broccoli © Madhur Jaffrey, 1998, is reproduced by permission of the author, c/o Rogers Coleridge & White, Ltd, 20 Powis Mews, London W11 1JN.

Dorling Kindersley would like to thank Toni Kay for design and Helen Blanchard for design assistance; Caroline Barty for food styling for photography; Claire Cross for editorial assistance; Jane Knott for proof-reading; and Sue Bosanko for the index.

Many thanks to the models
Catherine Chambers, Eleanor Chambers, Laura Chambers, Adam Jogee, Kamilah Jogee, Alexander Kay, Charlotte Kay, Richard Kay, and Eloise Newton.

Picture credits
Gettyone Stone Christopher Bissell jacket front br; David Oliver 4tl, 79b.
Rex Interstock Ltd 75br; Organic Picture Library 23br.
Telegraph Colour Library Ed Horn 26–27, 28–29, 30–31; Masterfile 34–35, 36–37, 38–39, 40–41.